THE TRAUMA WE DON'T TALK ABOUT

VOLUME 2

THE TRAUMA WE DON'T TALK ABOUT

TOOLS FOR LIVING AND LIFE-CHANGING
STORIES OF PRESERVATION, HEALING,
LOVE, AND ADVOCACY OF THE SELF

VOLUME 2

ANA MAEL

HELLO

I don't know who you are, but I hope by reading this book you will know you are not alone in trauma.

If you find one essay or poem that speaks to you, that you can relate to, let me know which one. I would like to hear from you.

Email me at ana@anamael.com

First Edition

Editor: Bryanne Salazar

Cover Design : Alex Kirby
Interior Design: Typeflow
Author Photo: Samuel Engelking

Print ISBN: 978-1-7388318-5-2
Ebook ISBN: 978-1-7388318-6-9
Audio ISBN: 978-1-7388318-7-6

This book is dedicated to my sons, my family, each of my clients, mentors, teachers, the precious faculty and colleagues at the Somatic Experiencing Institute, my friends, star seeds, earth angels, and ancestors, all of whom helped me awaken the power within myself and assisted me in doing the same for others.

This book is also dedicated to everyone who was robbed of their self-advocacy and truth in order to survive.

CONTENTS

INTRODUCTION

THIS BOOK BEGAN AS A JOURNAL IN WHICH I recorded personal experiences and thoughts as I worked through my own healing process and continued, later on, to help many in trauma recovery in my therapy office.

Now, I have compiled these personal writings into The Trauma We Don't Talk About series, with the intention of inspiring, empowering, and validating people with PTSD and trauma.

Each piece in this creative flash nonfiction collection is a tale of self-reliance, healing, the strength of the survival brain, and the wisdom of our trauma bodies. These stories encourage those who have experienced trauma to self advocate, give grace to their pain, and rediscover their thirst for life, while developing a sense of self-love — maybe for the first time in their life.

These essays are designed to evoke empathy, understanding, and also discomfort by challenging individuals and communities to reflect on their own trauma histories while also pursuing positive action to break the silence surrounding mental health and honest discussions of pain, as I did by reliving my trauma truth. It's time to start talking about it.

1

TRAUMA MIND

GOODBYE DIDN'T HAPPEN

WHAT'S LEFT INSIDE OF YOU WHEN YOU DON'T GET to say goodbye? When you had to flee and run away to literally save your life? When you were abruptly uprooted by your terrified parents, or left to survive all alone, or when you crossed the border, running and desperate to stay alive by making it to a safe house, what was left inside of you?

What happened to you then? When everyone who knew you was taken away from you, what was left of you? What were you left with?

How did you live when those necessary goodbyes didn't happen? When gentle send-offs weren't possible, when there were no hugs from friends, no holding of your hands, no arms to embrace you, no teary eyes, no kind words to wish you well? When there was no one to say, "Good luck on your journey; you can always come back"?

Your life is defined by that moment. The life before you fled and the life after. The life you had until the moment of exile and all that came after. Before displacement and after.

What happened after, and how did you survive? When

you never got your send-off into the world, the world never became a safe place. There were no people to come back to when the world became overwhelming. There was no safe haven. There was no refuge. The world became unsafe, an overwhelming space to live in, and a place from which you couldn't escape back into the safe hands of people who loved you.

Your nervous system remembers leaving in shame, with confusion, guilt, and fear. It remembers being exiled without friends or family. It remembers fleeing when the only thing you wanted to do was stay.

Where did you land? You lived between two worlds. The world you can never go back to and the overwhelming new world of uncertainty and loneliness. It's a place filled with insecurity.

It's a life divided into before and after you had to flee. From your land, into no one's land.

SCARED TO BE
BY YOURSELF

SOMETIMES, STAYING IN A TOXIC RELATIONSHIP IS less frightening than deciding to leave and just be by yourself. Instead, you've tenaciously tried to figure out everything you can about your toxic partner. You've pinpointed all of their needs, wishes, wants, patterns, likes, dislikes, triggers, yeses, and nos.

You know them well. You can even predict what they'll do before they can. Your detector is so precise and sensitive that it can sense all the layers of their being. You're on call and always waiting to meet their needs. But who is waiting for you when you decide to leave the relationship?

It's you. You get to stay with yourself, which is scary because you are someone you don't yet know. You are someone you lost, someone you abandoned. You could not name, nor do you know, your own needs, wishes, wants, patterns, likes, dislikes, triggers, yeses and nos.

They are deeply unknown to you, or once known and long forgotten. Who is that stranger you need to stay with now? Who are you and where do you find the energy to get to know yourself when you've invested everything in getting to know someone who made you abandon yourself in the first place?

That is why it's easier to stay in a toxic relationship than to leave and stay with yourself. It's not as lonely to sit with someone you know so well, even if they are toxic, as it is to sit with the unknown self.

LEFT OUT, LEFT BEHIND, LEFT ON THE SIDE

WHEN WE WERE ABANDONED IN THE PAST BY OUR parents, friends, or even our partner, we fell into an abyss of fear. That experience stays with us, and it causes us to fall into the same abyss of fear when we see someone leaving us in the present, even if all they're doing is going back home. The feeling of being left behind, of being left on our own, of not knowing what will happen to us next, is one we spend our lives trying to avoid.

The trauma body remembers pain. It also remembers the turmoil and shock from when we were abandoned without a choice. It remembers the intensity of grief and the heartbreak of being left. It remembers the realization that we didn't have a say in whether or not we were invited back, in whether or not we belonged.

We were left powerless and stuck in a place of waiting for others to decide. Left out, left behind, and left on the side. That is why we hate goodbyes. We can't stomach them. We avoid them, conveniently skipping them with our suddenly too-busy schedules. When we need to say goodbye to someone, we might feel confused and awkward.

The truth is, we simply don't want to be reminded of that state of abandonment.

What we can do now is to allow ourselves to say goodbye, and then intentionally notice how our day and routine continue. Maybe we can visit with friends for dinner, or go to the movies, or go shopping. We can notice how life goes on in the same space, and how different the aftermath of that goodbye feels now.

We can notice how someone we did say goodbye to follows up with us through texts and DMs. We can see that we were not abandoned, left out, left behind, or left on the side. We can realize that someone who left us physically in the present can still be in our lives, and that they will continue to be there for us if we each choose it.

Allow your body to feel this new and different sensation, that this is not the trauma state our survival brain remembers. It is a life full of reliable connections with others that we can look forward to.

IMPULSE

The impulse to help you erased me.

I stopped wanting. I stopped feeling.

I gave up my needs so I could serve yours.

Serving you led me to disappear.

I ceased to exist,
believing it was the only way to be with you.

YOU NO LONGER NEED WHAT YOU LEARNED AS A CHILD

A YOUNG CHILD CANNOT CHANGE THEIR PARENTS OR run away. A young child doesn't even know there's an option to call out for help. They don't yet have the tools to navigate life. But what that child does develop—over time and sub-consciously—are the tools for survival.

A child tries to protect their heart from deep emotional wounding by closing down their body. Human instinct tells them to protect themselves by bracing their bodies and restricting their breath.

As a child, you can't run away from a violent parent, so your survival wisdom helps you to protect your body by fully closing yourself into a shell. You do this to protect your heart from tremendous fear and pain by never allowing yourself to fully breathe.

What happens if this protective tool doesn't allow the trauma in your body to be released when you become an adult? It means you remain trapped in the memory of fear that you carried as a child.

Trauma is stuckness, and as an adult, you might still be stuck in that protective shell, braced and holding your breath, and safeguarding your heart as you did when you were a wise child.

You're an adult now, and you deserve to have adult tools for living, not the protective tools you had to use as a child. Many times, using those tools is the reason you still feel like a child, the reason you are still holding your breath and feeling powerless around others. What's tricky is that you might not even be aware that you are in a braced and closed-off state because it's the only state you know. It's the way you have held your body for the past couple of decades. It is your normal.

You stay stuck in this state because your trauma mind still feels like a helpless child, waiting for permission to become an adult, or waiting for someone to come and show you that it's okay to be an adult now.

So, if you have been waiting for permission, give yourself that permission now. If you have been waiting for someone to show you that it's okay to access your responsibility and your authority as an adult, follow my lead. Profound healing can start once you embrace adult tools for living. But first, you need to learn what those adult tools are, right? No one was there to teach you. The survival tools you do have, you developed on your own.

One tool is making sure your environment and the people you interact with are safe. If anyone makes you feel like you need to go into that familiar shell, to close yourself off and restrict your breath, then use that as a signal to tap into your toolbox. Make the choice to move toward safer, kinder people. Your second tool is movement. Learn to move your body through the free flow of expression as ecstatic dance, or any other free-form dance. In movement, the muscle memory of trauma gets softened and released. It's the same way with singing. Let the sound out.

A good therapist will guide you and teach you what you need in your toolbox in order to live a safe and normal life without bracing or holding your breath to survive. Once you acquire those tools and practice using them, softening and tenderness in your mind and body, along with a sense of agency and being an adult will follow.

HOW DO YOU HOLD MY SHAME?

How do you hold my shame
when you entertain?
When you casually chat?
When you're charming others?

What about at night?
When you can't keep yourself agile and upright?
Is my shame taking space in your mind?
It was yours from the start, never mine.

It resides in you. You know that, right?
I wonder how you hold yourself at night.
Do you sweat? Does your heart race?
Pills never helped. You know you can't run away.

You beg for the day to start, so shame can drift away.
You bury yourself in work,
though you know it doesn't help.
The shame inside of you will always echo
the misery and harm you left behind.

I bet you are still breaking hearts;
nothing else can come from your toxic,
narcissistic skin, but only sins.

INNER CRITIC

YOUR INNER CRITIC IS THE MOST FRIGHTENED AND most demanding part of you. It's so afraid of rejection and terrified of feeling judged and humiliated that it demands nothing but perfection and overcompensation from you.

That critical, cutting, and cruel voice in your head that tells you what you must do or how you should have done it — while pointing out each of your faults — is actually the voice of a terrorized child. Pay attention to the tone of that voice. It might sound like the voice of your mother, your father, or an abusive sibling.

That's because the scared part of you took their threatening voice and internalized it. It modeled that internal voice from the outside, so it could demand perfection from you in order to protect you from being harmed again. That voice may sound like an adult, but ask yourself, when did this inner critic arrive? Usually, it develops between the ages of eight and twelve. It is nothing more than a scared child, trying to protect themself from harm.

The inner critic is both a trauma response and a self-protection mechanism. If you weren't perfect — if you were too loud, or didn't have good manners, or weren't routinely the best at everything — you likely faced a great amount of shame and hurt from your family of origin.

Pay attention to your inner critic when it arises and say to it:

I know you sound like the person who shamed me, but now I recognize that you are my child self, who's terrified that we will be shamed again. I'm an adult now, and I'm learning how to self-advocate and set up boundaries. I know that no one will harm us. I know you want to protect me. You can go rest and let me figure out how to do this, without being perfect. This time, we can mess up and we will be ok.

SO, HOW CAN I NOT KNOW?

IN TRAUMA, YOU KEEP YOURSELF SAFE BY MAKING sure you know everything, and yet, how can you be expected to know what you were never taught? How can you know what a normal relationship is when you have never experienced one? How can you know the name for a feeling when you've never heard it named? In trauma, "I don't know" means "I will not survive." How can you *not* know everything and stay alive?

You'll notice a physical response when you realize you are allowed to not know. Not knowing is a learning curve for every trauma survivor, but it's worth the climb to reach a place where you feel safer. Not knowing is a place of trust, of trusting that someone else will know instead of you, and that this someone is reliable and trustworthy. It's a space of expansion.

How did your family, your lineage, handle not knowing? Did your ancestors have the luxury of not knowing? You do.

WHAT THEY WANT
US TO BELIEVE

ABUSE, WHICH INCLUDES EMOTIONAL ABUSE, MICRO-aggressions, bullying at work, abuse of power by your boss or another authority figure, toxic parenting, or a sibling verbally attacking you, produces an enormous amount of shame, which inhibits your ability for self-expansion and social growth.

This shame is so powerful because it creates a cyclical, inhibitory response in the nervous system that tells you to avoid connection because of the fear of that connection causing more shame. Like a dog chasing its own tail, your shame feeds your belief that you are unworthy of connection, and that lack of connection proves your shame right.

Your abuser imposed the belief that something about you is inherently wrong and toxic to others. These are your abuser's thoughts inside of you, not yours. How did they get there? It can start with subtle comments that insult your intelligence, your abilities, your career, your looks, and more. These thoughts burrow into your brain and impact your beliefs about yourself.

I want you to know that you are inherently worthy, and healthy people will respect, celebrate, and value you. All the toxicity and wrongness that was thrown at you belongs to your abuser, not you. They saw their flaws, and the only way they knew how to rid themselves of their shame was to project it onto you.

You belong with others, and you are worthy of connection. If shame or fear of embarrassment arises while you are trying to connect, I want you to pause. Remind yourself that this is exactly how your bully wanted you to feel. Remember that they wanted you to believe that you are unworthy of connection. Then, in spite of your abuser, try to make a connection. Even if you embarrass yourself, even if it is messy and awkward, you can self-advocate and rebuild your confidence.

WHY DID I REPULSE SO MANY?

WAS IT MY ETHNICITY? MY GENDER? MY REFUGEE status? The fact that I was homeless? Was it because I was an immigrant, or a farm worker? Why did I repulse so many?

I know why.

That repulsion came from a place of disgust inside of my oppressor's body, knowing what they did, or what they didn't do but could have done. It was their gut speaking up. Seeing my mistreatment reminded my abusers of their wrongness, of the inhumane treatment they were capable of. This is a hard truth to witness about oneself. Their body registered that disgust, but not their mind.

Their repulsion was not because of me, but because of what they did to me and to people like me. I was mirroring back the crimes they committed. Their body was releasing all of the stored disgust inside of them. Unwilling to acknowledge the true cause of their disgust, they directed it back at me.

Still, their body knew. It was never about me. It was what

festered inside of them. Disgust at their own wrongness, not mine. They were enraged by how filthy they felt, and yet they all believed they were noble and acting with a righteous purpose.

SELF-PUNISHMENT
IS PROTECTION

SELF-HARM, SELF-SABOTAGE, SELF-ALIENATION, self-judgment, and self-destruction are what your abuser wants to see you do to yourself. When your abuser destroys your spirit, it looks like your spirit is destroying itself, all on its own. That's exactly how the sadist wants you to be, lost in the madness of pain and self-punishment.

Everything coming from your abuser subconsciously leads to self-harm. It's as if by hurting yourself, you say to your abuser, "Don't touch me. I'm capable of harming myself now, so you don't have to. You showed me well. I will do it better than you, as long as you don't come close to me. Just leave me alone."

In a way, self-destructive impulses are an attempt to protect you from the pain of your abuser. If you protect yourself from being harmed again by them, then you have a sense of control over the pain you receive from yourself. It's a protective trauma response.

When emotional pressure reaches a peak inside of your body and there's no one to turn to, the buildup of pain from blame and guilt is released through self-harm. It's a painful trauma response and an even more painful trauma remedy.

If this is happening to you, I want to acknowledge that you are doing your best to protect yourself. There is no shame in that. This is purely your survival instinct and incredible intelligence taking action to keep you alive, even though it can look like self-destruction from the outside.

Who gets to judge you and your actions? Your desire to lessen your pain is understandable, and it is a reflection of the seriousness of the abuse you've faced.

What you need to know is that you are not alone and there are people who can help you. The sadistic abuser wants you to think you're alone, but I promise you're not.

A healthier release will come by reaching out to safe people or to one safe person. By doing this, the body finds new sources of support, and the impulse to hurt yourself will dissipate.

Self-harm comes from a place of deep isolation. Healing begins when you reach out to your support system—a friend, a therapist, or a school counselor—and when you know you're not alone when that emotional pressure builds.

Find out if you are in relationship
with a narcissist or a sociopath:
ptsdtraumarecovery.com/am-i-with-narcissist-quiz/

SHAME

IN TRAUMA, YOU LIVE IN THE SHADOW OF SHAME. IT never leaves you. It's sticky and glues itself to your being. Shame was dumped over you, and you continued to wear it, never allowing it to wash away. I wore so much shame, paired with tears and a familiar sense of loneliness, believing this wrongness was mine.

I really believed it was mine. I trusted what my abusers, government, and society said. I never questioned it. They made me believe they were better than me, and I cloaked myself in the shame they projected onto me. No amount of detoxing, cleansing, or retreats could remove it from me.

The younger you are when you are shamed, the more petrified the shame becomes, hardening into your identity. This shame becomes a silent, unseen building block in your body's structure. You cannot run away from shame, jump over it, or hide from it. Eventually, it always overtakes you, and the younger you are when it finds you, the longer your shadow of shame looms.

It follows you into your old age. It sticks with you, screams at you, digs its dirty fingernails into you. The more you try to wash it away, the more it wraps around you. Eventually, it finds its way inside of you, infiltrating each cell. As it penetrates your being, it begins to speak louder and louder each passing day.

You wish for the shame to shrink, subside, or fade away, but it's always there. You wish for a rainy day so that, maybe, the sticky shame can wash away and, at least until tomorrow, so you can take a breath and have a bit of rest.

WHAT IS MISSING
IN ABUSE?

PROTECTION IS WHAT'S MISSING IN ABUSE, NOT LOVE.
Abuse can happen from a place of love. A parent may believe
hitting their child to make them behave is an act of love.
Protection is what's missing, protection of the child, protection of their human rights, protection of their boundaries,
and protection of their dignity.

Who didn't protect you? Who wasn't there for you? Was
it your mother, your father, your grandparents, your school,
your neighbors, your siblings, your relatives, your government,
your country—who could have protected you and didn't?

LONELY

Lonely, lonely, lonely—age five.

Lonely, lonely, lonely—age eight.

Lonely, lonely, lonely—age fourteen.

Lonely, lonely, lonely—age fifteen.

Lonely, lonely, lonely—age seventeen.

Lonely, lonely, lonely—age eighteen.

Lonely, lonely, lonely—age nineteen.

Lonely, lonely, lonely—age twenty.

Lonely, lonely, lonely—age twenty-one.

Lonely, lonely, lonely—age twenty-two.

Lonely, lonely, lonely—age forty-five.

Then your eyes met and welcomed mine,

and I saw myself for the first time.

FAMILY SILENCE

Nothing makes you feel so wrong and so
unworthy of existence, like family silence.

It encourages the mistreatment of other
family members and allows the punitive
system of that "good" neighbor or coach.

Family silence makes you feel like you
deserve to be hurt and humiliated.

It teaches you that speaking your
truth will be costly for you.

It teaches you that you are unworthy of protection.

It teaches you that speaking out means you
will not be welcomed back, not ever.

Family silence.

PACK YOUR THINGS NOW!

I WAS FOURTEEN WHEN MY PARENTS SUDDENLY TOLD me to pack what I needed for a few days.

"We have to leave!" they yelled. I looked confused. I was absorbing what I was just told when my mother screamed in my face, "We will be killed! We need to run away!"

Why? I didn't do anything wrong, I thought. I didn't want to pack. I wanted to stay there. At least I deserved to say goodbye. I wasn't leaving until my friends came and said goodbye to me and wished me good luck!

Grabbed by the elbow, I was pushed down our condo stairs, out the door and into the car, pressed between my two sisters and our bags. Did I matter so little? Was this my life?

I didn't say or hear any goodbyes. I wanted to run away. Where were my friends? In my mind, I wanted to scream, *You cannot take me away from my home! I am not fleeing into displacement! Can anyone, someone, please just show up, send me off, and say goodbye?*

I was about to flee from my home. I stared through the car window, hoping my friends would show up and see me. They didn't know we were running away, and I didn't know if I would ever come back.

I told myself that maybe my friends didn't care about me. At least that's what I pretended. It was a less devastating way to make sense of all the changes that had happened in just twenty minutes.

I pleaded for my parents to let me stay where I belonged, to tell me why this was happening. I wanted them to just let me just stay with my friends. I had done nothing wrong.

I just wanted to be stuck—like the roots of a tree—in the place I knew, because where I was about to go was the vastness of the unknown, where survival meant having no identity, where I would spend a decade hiding in shame. I wanted to be stuck, or at least, to hear someone say to me, "Goodbye and good luck."

WHY DIDN'T YOU STAND UP?

MY PARENTS NEVER STOOD UP FOR ME, SO I MADE myself believe I was deserving of everyone's insults.

ABOUT TO LOSE
MY MIND

Having lost your mind is painless.
It's a place of release, no thoughts, no
meaning, no heaviness.
It's almost carefree and liberating to lose your
mind. Mindlessness is a restful place to be.

The place where I was *about* to lose
my mind was the worst.
It was a place of constant anticipation.
A place of turmoil, anguish, and the deepest isolation.
A place of fear where time didn't exist,
where people didn't exist.
Where I didn't exist.

A place where the only sound was the
terrified cries inside my body.
A place where the next hour felt so far away,
and the next day was too overwhelming to imagine.
It was a place of constant inner listening,
where I was just *about* to lose my mind.
Where I was *about* to lose it all.

BEGINNING OF THE ABUSE

I TOOK MY ABUSER'S DESCRIPTION OF ME AS MY REALity, and the only truth about me. That is how much they distorted my mind so they could have full control over me.

Don't let anyone tell you what is true about yourself. Trust your experiences, trust your reality, trust your facts, trust your emotions, and trust your humanity. When you start to doubt yourself, that's the beginning of abuse.

PROMISED TO WAIT

IN REPETITIVE ABUSE, MANY THINGS ARE CERTAIN. YOU know how it will end. You know how it will leave you feeling, the taste that will linger in your mouth, and the smell of your pain.

A feeling of craziness often comes, not from the end result of abuse, but from the uncertainty of waiting, from the anticipation of the promised abuse.

Promises like, "Wait until I come home."

You were promised harm that could come at any day, any hour, any minute, or any second. You just needed to wait for it. You didn't know when it was coming, and that space of waiting became a space of losing yourself, a space where all you could hear were your fearful, frantic thoughts.

It was a space where no one—no matter how empathetic they tried to be—could understand, unless they lived in it too. Survivors of trauma can understand, but others can't. This is why waiting around for someone, a friend, or a doctor, or a meeting to start, or standing in any sort of line, can activate your trauma.

Communicate your need for others to be on time, or find a support buddy, or keep yourself busy with a book or podcast. Don't allow anyone to dismiss your experience of how it felt to be in that space of promised waiting. Don't let them minimize your need not to wait. The threat of abuse waiting for you was real. It was the truth. It was yours, and it was hell.

MY PARTNER THE SOCIOPATH

You commend me for getting myself together.
As if I'm an embarrassment when I'm seen with you.
As if I'm dirt that smudges your
picture-perfect appearance.
As if it shames you to be connected to me.
As if I'm somehow less than you.

And even if I get myself together, for whom
should I be seen, for whom should I be?
You isolated me and broke me down, all
so you could glare over me,
so you could be aroused by watching me wither away.

Know this, my presence will always
overshadow your high-paid publicity,
and your sadistic mind will always sizzle with jealousy.

You fear being displaced and dismissed by others.
It's your constant fear that you will
be discovered as a fraud,
and that all of the inadequacy in the core
of your being will finally be seen.

It's your awareness of who you are
that offends you so much,
so you push me down to try and rise above me.
You made me the projection of your
inner disgust and toxic shame,
to replace what you know about yourself.

You may abuse me so that I'm not a constant
reminder of what you can't achieve,
but this hole of inadequacy inside of you is sucking you in.
No matter how many achievements you make or
how much money you add to your bank accounts,
that shame keeps eating you alive.

Presence comes from the backbone, and
that is something you can't acquire.
It comes from the soul. It comes from pure love and grace.
Publicity and money can buy you pretense,
but presence is something that can never
form inside of your empty core.

FEAR OF SILENCE

THE COMPULSIVE IMPULSE TO FILL THE EMPTY space in a conversation comes from a deep fear of silence. In abuse, that dome of silence means your perpetrator—someone who has power over you—also has complete control over you.

In that single, silent moment, in that pregnant pause, you know something harmful is about to happen to you. You can neither control it nor escape it. You just know it's coming. Silence is the moment right before the abuse begins, and silence is the shame and shock that fills you after the abuse is done.

If you meet someone who talks a lot without taking a pause, someone who is constantly trying to fill the void, they have most likely experienced abuse. Look at that person with more compassion, love, and care, and let them fill the void of silence. Let them talk.

DEPRIVED

WHEN YOU COME FROM DEPRIVATION, YOU DISCI-pline yourself to live an ascetic life. Being shamed for having basic needs or wants evokes deep feelings of rejection in a child. When you are rejected, you don't belong, and for a child, belonging to their family is their main source of safety.

So you learned that in order to feel safe, you needed to be-long, and that asking for your needs could provoke rejection from others. This is how you conditioned yourself to never ask for anything. You learned it was better to deprive yourself of any need than to be deprived of belonging and safety.

MASTER OVERRIDERS

TRAUMA SURVIVORS ARE MASTER OVERRIDERS.

Once, I knew I had been touched without my consent by a medical professional. I felt discomfort and awkwardness. Yet, I kept talking and overriding my sense of unease, just so I wouldn't make other people uncomfortable—including the medical professional who had made me feel that way. Yes, the person who had just unethically touched me, I kept quiet so I would not embarrass them. Wow!

Even as an adult woman, the scared child within me was still leading. The child who made it her fault when other people left her feeling confused, uneasy, or ashamed. I was conditioned to believe I deserved inhumane treatment and that I couldn't and shouldn't expect better from people.

I blamed myself, never conceiving of blaming them or holding them accountable. I truly believed something was wrong with me, and that this was how people like me were supposed to be treated. I had very little regard for self-protection, and nearly no understanding or sense of my worth or what I deserved.

Even after a lengthy time as an adult, I had the tendency to override my experiences and to place a higher value on others, even those who saw me as less. This was my programmed response, even when the person I was deferring to lacked a moral compass or competency.

This changed when I promised myself that, moving forward, every time I felt a subtle notch of discomfort or awkwardness stemming from someone else, I would stop time. I would stop the planet.

I would give that small, unprotected girl within me—the one who learned to silence her discomfort and override her instincts—the full protection she never had. I would use my voice to stand up for her. I would not be quiet. I especially would not override my confusion, embarrassment, or anger to make the person who caused it feel more comfortable.

ARE YOU A BACKUP SINGER SUPPRESSING YOUR OWN POTENTIAL?

ARE YOU THE ONE WHO SUPPRESSES AND MINIMIZES your own potential? Are you the one who never works to your full capacity? You know you have it, you can feel it in your bones, in your intelligent, quick mind, and yet you hide it, allowing others to show their acumen, even though they're clearly less competent than you.

You yield to them and walk to the back of the room. You live as a backup singer, always allowing someone else to shine in the spotlight, never yourself. Do you wonder why? Who suffers if you show your true potential? Who would feel uncomfortable or angry if you start showing up and taking space?

Growing up, we often learn to diminish ourselves to avoid shame. You might have had a jealous sibling or friend, or a parent who would always praise their less adept child while telling you to not show off or demonstrate your gifts, so you didn't appear cocky or arrogant.

You were hushed and minimized. You might have even been punished for your intelligence or saying something smart. That conditioning and taming sticks with you as an adult. You keep yielding, allowing others to outshine you. You keep giving space to people with less talent. You keep acquiescing so that less capable people have the chance to earn even more money than you.

It isn't even their fault. They have nothing to do with your childhood conditioning. Ask yourself, who actually suffers when you don't live up to your potential? You. You are the one who suffers, not the people you keep allowing to take your space.

You don't need your parents' permission—or anyone else's—to take up space. You own it yourself. You can unleash all the potency and intelligence you've kept stifled inside of you. You might be surprised by how many healthy people there are around you, people who would like to be with you on the center stage in the musical of your life. You might be surprised by how many people cheer for you in this phase of your life.

Surround yourself with cheerleaders, not jealous people or those who kill your light so they can shine. That was never your burden to carry. No, you are allowed to light up and shine.

UNHIDE YOURSE_F

Don't give up.

Unhide your face,
unsilence your voice,
unshame your presence;
shame was never in your essence.

Unwrong the wrongness you feel about yourself,
unsoil the dirt you feel on your face,
they were given in pettiness by others.

Ungive-up on yourself and see your true spark.
Hear your rich voice and witness your inherent worth.
You were never supposed to hide!
You are the most precious gem in my life.

You are my pulse.
You are the one who is ferocious and
brave, gracious and kind.

Unhide your face,
unsilence your voice.

Put the burden of shame where it belongs,
outside of your skin,
off your face,
out of your voice,
far from your presence.

You can now take space.
You can be seen.
You are a treasure,
so unhide your gifts.
You mean so much to me.

Yes, you are important,
and yes, you do exist
inside of me.

DIVINE LOVE

Perpetrator: You! Stay down; only I can shine!
My glory comes only when I keep
you pressed to the ground.
Don't you dare look up! You want freedom?
You want to fly above the ground?
Ha! Stay down!
Only I can shine.
You want to expand? Show your smartness all around?
No! No one will outshine me or darken my light!
You will only look down!
I will place you into this box of mine.
I am the ceiling above your head now.
You won't break free from me, and if you try,
I will keep pressing you deeper down!

Me: Oh, I am looking down.
Press me! Press me, press me more, press me down.
I know you know how.
But you cannot take my light.
You think you have power over me?
I am looking at the ground, but only to survive.

There is a magical place I always drift away to
when you think you are putting me into
that box on your command.
Press me, press me, press me down!
You will never take away my spite.

I drift away to an expansive place.
My soul is flying above that box you think you control.

My spirit is free, there is a bounty of
beauty of which you will never see.
Every time you think you are pressing me into the ground,
I fly above you, into the sky.
It is a place full of grace,
where I am loved by all my divine friends.

And just so you know, in a single second,
I can turn into an expansive beast,
filled with protective anger.
I can grab you by your neck, pull you down,
and stare into your contemptuous eyes.
I can stamp down upon your face with
my foot and watch you dissipate.

I will look into your eyes and see you,
pressed deep into the ground.
How does it feel now?
Look at the anger in my eyes when you are on the ground.
Do you feel fear crawling up your face?

Tell me, in this moment, can your soul drift away?
Can you protect yourself from this stream of hate?
Do you have any divine friends? Can you
find consolation in the divine?
Can you be embraced with pure love?
Can you feel the hatred from others and
know that it can never spoil your pristine essence?

Can you become so expansive, so filled with grace,
and — at the same time — feel hatred
pressing you from the outside?
No?

I am not surprised. That ability comes from the soul.
That is the divine you will never find.
I will always outshine you with love.

You can never press me deep enough into the ground.
I transformed the hatred I witnessed in your eyes
into my strength and pristine love.
I know I can press you down. You deserve to suffer and die.
But I will let you live in the desperation of constant fear
that your inadequacy will be discovered.
I want you to linger in your anguish.
Let that inner shame eat you alive.

Yes, I will outshine you,
no matter how deep you keep
pressing me into the ground.

LACK OF CHOICE

YOUR ABUSER DESTROYS YOUR SENSE OF SELF-worth so that you depend on them completely. This creates codependency. Your abuser can be a controlling, authoritarian parent, a jealous lover, or even a manipulative family member.

Your abilities, your values, your sense of self and your agency did not exist when you were raised or lived with someone who had power over you. Don't think of abuse as only a physical experience. Abuse can be covert, including emotionally blaming and constantly condemning you.

When you live a codependent life, where someone else defines your day, your choices, your likes and dislikes, you lose your sense of autonomy and agency.

The sad part is, your abuser never works in your best interest when they are making your decisions, choices, and plans. You are nothing but an extension of their self-loathing.

This is the essence of abuse. You are left dependent upon someone else's opinions with a destroyed sense of self. Interestingly, this lack of choice is also the reason many people learn to manipulate others.

This behavior isn't born out of malice; rather, it is a way for the victim to get their needs met. Many people who learn to manipulate were never given a chance to make decisions for themselves, let alone consider that they had the right to make their own choices.

This is what abuse does. It deprives victims of the knowledge that they don't need anyone's permission or approval to make choices in their lives.

2

ISOLATION AND THE LOST SELF

ISOLATION AND PTSD

ISOLATION IS A PLACE WHERE LONELINESS, PAIN, shame, and self-judgment are met with the belief that you have to experience all of these states on your own. It's you against the world.

To leave isolation behind, you have to do the math and calculate how many people are around you. Then, you might realize that you're not alone. From the people you live with, to the people you meet in support groups, at work, in a coffee shop, or at a bookstore, there are people all around you. Count them. They didn't live through what you did. They will never know exactly what it was like for you, but thankfully, they don't have to.

They can still root for you, feel genuine emotions for you, and honestly want to be with and even talk to you. Notice these people every day. Feel a small sense of gratitude for everyone you meet. By noticing the people around you, you're moving yourself out of the isolation of PTSD. You're never really alone, even if no one else you know went through what you did.

STOP TRYING

TRYING IS THE EFFORT TO SURVIVE. TRYING TO MOVE through the day, trying to hide how much you are struggling, trying to get through a meeting without having a panic attack, trying to breathe through dinner so you don't run away, trying to bite your cheeks so you don't erupt with rage.

All of it is trying. In a trauma body, trying comes from a place of constant struggle. In the back of your mind, there is always the insinuation that how hard you try, things will still be the same. Yet, you keep trying. Living in that head-space throughout your life brings enormous exhaustion into your body.

You want to live. You want to survive, and that drive pushes you to try. You place more and more expectations and demands on yourself, which ultimately leaves you in despair. Yet, you keep trying. This is how life feels for people with trauma and PTSD, and this constant state of effort, despair, and trying to survive can last for decades.

At some point in my own healing, I altered my narrative. I substituted *trying* with *learning*. I told myself: *I will learn to get through the day. I will learn to share my struggle, and someone will help me. I will learn my only responsibility is to meet my needs today. I will learn.*

Just focus on that word, *learn*. It's airy, fluid, less pushy, and less demanding. Learning allows for the possibility of error and provides you wiggle room to figure things out. It puts less survival pressure on your nervous system. There are fewer expectations and less of a need to keep up with everyone. When you live with trauma, you need to learn how to live again.

You need to replace your trauma reactions with conscious responses. Life is now a school you are attending, and you are a student who needs to learn the basics of normal living. When you are constantly trying, exuding effort, you are back in the trenches of war, lost in trauma mode.

Instead, you need to pause and invite curiosity into every single task you do, day by day. Feel it in your body. Notice how it feels. Is it less heavy, is it more freeing, does it offer more space for exploration? Allow your body to feel the possibility of learning.

Then, bring this page to your therapist to discuss it with them, and make a plan to learn new pathways of safety and thriving.

LISTENING

I was never misunderstood.

To be misunderstood, you need to be privileged enough to be listened to in the first place.

My voice was never listened to.

THE SADIST IN ME

I DEMANDED A HIGH-LEVEL OF PERFORMANCE FROM myself, demanded constant hypervigilance, and maintained my own readiness—for anything—at a moment's notice. I was alert and ready to aim and shoot, twenty-four seven.

Of all the wars I lived through, this inner war was, by far, the worst. I couldn't displace myself from it, even decades after my life continued in peace.

WHAT HELPS?

DEPRESSION IS SCARED OF MOVEMENT BECAUSE IT feeds off stuckness. So, move your body. Dance it out, walk it out, sound it out, write it out, sing it out, talk it out.

Just move and get it out. Movement and sound. Repeat this every day, or every hour, if necessary. Dance can be a powerful medicine in trauma recovery. Commit to it and make it a ritual, as if your life depends on it. In a way, it does.

Depression likes loneliness, but you deserve happiness and connection. Look for support, schedule a session with a therapist, spend time with animals, find someone you can sit with and process your trauma, move your trauma narrative out of your body. Find a place where you can be with people, even when you don't need to talk or don't feel like sharing. Just get out and move with others.

CONSENT

HOW LONG DID YOU STICK WITH SOMETHING YOU didn't like? Did uncomfortable or unpleasant things happen to you, but you convinced yourself that you were supposed to like them?

When did touch become unpleasant? When did sex become something painful that you were somehow supposed to like? When did a joke become shameful or hurtful, yet you laughed along with others?

Many assaults happen right at the moment that we think we gave in because we didn't say anything, and somehow that means we gave consent. Our survival brains are conditioned to do anything to endure, and the moment your nervous system kicks into survival mode, you won't even consider saying, "I don't like that."

That's why so many people feel shame around not doing or saying anything to resist, and just going along with a hurtful or humiliating situation. Please know you didn't consent to harassment or abuse. Your nervous system went along with it because you were trained by your parents, your society, and your culture to put up with it, and your survival brain reacted by going into freeze or appeasement mode.

In that moment, your body didn't have a choice, and your conscious mind didn't know you could have a choice in the first place. Recovery starts when you ingrain it into your system that your human right is to have a choice when it comes to your body and mind. Then, you have the right and responsibility to communicate that choice out loud when things become even a tiny, tiny bit off for you. If you feel confusion, that's usually the first sign that someone just

The Trauma We Don't Talk About – *Volume 2*

crossed your boundaries. Even feeling a tiny micro-bit off or confused is enough of a reason for you to speak out.

You don't need to tolerate or appease, nor do you need to put up with something that takes you—even slightly—from a place of safety to a place of discomfort, confusion, harm, abuse, and silence.

CAN YOU LOOK PEOPLE IN THE EYES?

THE REASON YOU AVOID LOOKING PEOPLE IN THE eyes might be because you are afraid of the expression you will meet, or what you will see. The trauma brain remembers seeing an expression of rejection, contempt or burden in someone's eyes, and now you subconsciously avert your gaze from others to avoid that feeling.

Your eyes are afraid of what they will see and how you will feel when you are seen by others. Unfortunately, many times in the past, when someone's eyes met yours, you saw annoyance, frustration, anger, rage, or contempt. Your eyes don't want to look into anyone else's and see that again. Why would they? They are scared and tremendously tired.

PTSD LIVES ON
THE OTHER SIDE

PTSD FEELS LIKE LIVING YOUR LIFE ON THE OPPOSITE side of the border. It's as if there's a line between you and everyone else. The entire world is happening across that line. The border is fenced and guarded, and you are not permitted to cross it. Everyone else can live there, just not you.

You have no energy left inside of you to do anything but look at how good life is on the other side, in this so-called Promised Land, while you're stuck here, in the Land of Isolation. Here is a land where nothing can grow, where nothing is left, not even animals, where there is no sound or movement.

It's a land of isolated silence, except for the chatter of your constant thoughts. A land of the cursed, or the punished, you might think. You still might not know why you have been punished, why you are here. It's as if someone just dropped you and left you there for no reason.

In this parched and desolate landscape you look over the line to see how everyone continues to live. You see the families living their lives, playing with their kids, people happily walking their dogs, going to work or going about their day. It seems as if everyone there has a purpose and a sense of belonging. You feel a desperate longing to be with them, but it's as if you're frozen and stuck on this side, all alone.

You are on the PTSD side. Nothing, neither your legs, nor your arms, nor your mind can move you across that line. Yet your heart cries, wanting to be there and belong with others. It's a state of deep powerlessness.

For some reason, all the people you see across that line

feel a universe apart, and yet they could practically be sitting next to you, calling you to join them on their walk, or grab a coffee, or play a game together. Or perhaps they're just a click away, in a workshop, or a support group, or an online session with a therapist.

The reality is, that even though you feel alone, you might not actually be. Perhaps you have a family member who wants to help. Notice them. Perhaps you meet a kind cashier at the convenience store. They are truly a hand away, next to you, not across that line. You may not believe it, but you need to allow your eyes to see it. You have survived things that are so much harder than reaching out to others. This may be difficult, but it will not be devastating.

You start by eliminating that walled-off border PTSD created, and then you take the first steps away from isolation and toward togetherness and belonging with the people close to you.

IS GETTING SICK ALLOWED?

AFTER THE ONSET OF ANY SYMPTOMS OF SICKNESS or pain, you might immediately feel panic and despair. Your body jumps into a trauma state because it remembers that getting sick in your family wasn't allowed or accepted as a normal part of being alive.

Were you fully nurtured by your parents when you had menstrual pain, migraines, IBS, or otherwise felt unwell? Or did your parents seem burdened just because you got sick? Did you see the annoyance on their face? A look of disbelief? Were you dismissed when you said you weren't feeling well—as if it was nothing—or were you mocked?

Perhaps your parents expressed a great deal of anxiety when you were sick, which made you decide it was easier to take care of yourself because you didn't want to be scolded for making your mother "sick and worried," even though you were the one who was sick and worried.

How dare you experience illness? Were you even allowed to show symptoms of being sick? That's a terrifying place to be for a child or adolescent, to feel unwell and not have anyone to care for you. It's a place of fear, loneliness, and pain.

What you carry from this neglectful conditioning is the inability to ever get sick. It's not even an option because you would feel like a burden to your partner, friend, or even your doctor. You hide and minimize your symptoms, or ignore them completely, because getting sick was never accepted in your childhood family.

Your parents made you feel so desperate and lonely, that even now, as an adult, you might hide your condition or diagnosis, believing sickness is shameful, as if it's some plague you carry. Annoying everyone around you with your health problems isn't an option, either. Many trauma survivors have died alone in their beds with terminal illnesses, hiding the fact that they were sick from everyone.

Even if you don't say a word about it, your sickness may cause you to spiral. When you first experience symptoms, you might go straight into hypochondriac mode, Googling down a rabbit hole, diagnosing yourself into full panic mode, making you feel as if you're literally dying.

Your inability to be unwell as a child might cause you to go to the extreme end of healthiness as an adult, where you maintain a strict, organic, toxin – and germ-free diet, and live in a sterile environment, because of your anxiety about staying healthy.

In normal families, when you get sick you are nurtured, taken care of, loved, helped, and supported as long as you need it, and you receive follow-up care once you're back on your feet again.

You aren't abandoned, judged, shamed, mocked, or dismissed for being sick. Never. You were supposed to have a nurturing hand to hold you and tend to you when you were unwell. Getting sick is not—and never was—a shameful thing.

REMINDED HOW WORTHLESS YOU ARE

DESPERATELY WANTING TO BE RECOGNIZED AND approved of by others is the easiest path to self-abandonment and internal resentment. When you're in a toxic environment, everything you do—all the serving and effort to prove your worth—is useless.

Toxic people will always remind you of how worthless you are. The way out of this is to step away from them. You don't need their approval. You can move away from them and place yourself amongst people who routinely offer kind words, encouragement, validation, and respect.

Only when your efforts are matched—when you are valued, respected, and seen as a human being—do you offer your help, service, and the investment of your time.

WHY YOU FEEL STUCK

EVERYTHING IN YOU WANTS TO CONNECT WITH people, and simultaneously, everything in you wants to protect yourself from people. The energy inside of you feels like having one foot on the gas so you can accelerate toward connection, where you can belong and be loved, and having the other foot on the brake to prevent human connection because, in the past, connection caused you pain and heartbreak.

The human engine in you, with these conflicting energies, doesn't know what to do. This engine keeps accelerating and braking, roaring and squealing, sucking all the gas, all of your vital energy, from you. You might go in a circle, screeching tires leaving black-rubber donut marks on the pavement, working so hard to move fast, though you're not actually moving anywhere.

This push and pull energy keeps you stuck. Your nervous system doesn't know what to do with it. Does it move forward to connect, or run away from connection? It wants to join others, and it wants to run away at the same time.

Your cognitive mind and your soul don't know why you feel this anguish, why you can't fix this contradictory state. Your whole body is braced and silent. There is no movement toward people or away from them.

This is stuckness, and it's the most common trauma response to being hurt by people, and yet still needing to be loved and to give love. It's also the reason you struggle to maintain relationships, and the reason why you might hop from one partner to another.

These contradictory energies create a fear of commitment and intimacy, while leaving you longing for connection.

Outside of relationships, it can manifest as wanting to start a business, publish a book, or follow your dreams, and yet not being able to do anything about it except planning. Execution and completion never follow until you begin to heal.

DON'T BE ANYONE'S SHADOW

In pleasing everyone, I disappeared from existence.

No one noticed I vanished,
even though they were walking beside me,
continuing to talk about themselves, over and over again.

No one noticed my absence
because they never even noticed my presence.

UNTIL I DIE, I HAVE TO STAY IN THE SAME PLACE

THERE IS NO MIDDLE GROUND IN TRAUMA. WHEN someone says something will be a certain way, you don't question it. You don't even think you could question it. You have no liberty or freedom to question others, or to think for a moment that what you're hearing is bullshit.

Likewise, your place of employment feels as if it's the only place where you should, or even could, ever work. Not only do you have to be there, it's where you're obliged to stay because someone gave you that job. You feel like they did you a favor and that you're indebted to them because you earned a paycheck. You'll be paying that debt off forever.

With this attitude, you're placed at a desk, and someone else gets to decide your destiny. This kind of thinking makes you someone to pity, not an employee who provides their skills, knowledge, talent, labor, and time in return for their paycheck.

When it comes to making a choice for family vacations or reunions, you automatically follow what others decide, including where, how, when, and with whom. That uncle you can't stand? He's coming. The cruise your mother wants to take? You're going, even though you get desperately seasick. There's no middle ground where you can evaluate, change your mind, change your initial plans, communicate your own decisions, or even negotiate to make a mutual agreement. These aren't options in your mind.

You feel stuck where you are, obediently compromising and following others. It feels like you have to stay in this position until you die. This lack of power comes from your trauma body. The truth is that no one, not a micromanaging boss or snarky co-worker, a partner, a toxic circle of friends, toxic family members, or the place where you live can take your power from you. The truth is, you're not stuck. Trauma is stuck in your body.

MISSING A LIFE

IMAGINE THIS: SUMMER DAYS, LIVE MUSIC AT THE BAR, friends happily chatting, the wind in your hair, the sun warming your bones, your toes in the sand, a sway in your hips, sensuality in the air, parties until dawn, a celebration of milestones met.

You miss all of that, even though you might be right there, with the music in your ears, your toes in the sand, and friends dancing around you. You don't absorb, live, or even notice the good things in life. What you don't miss is your constant, simmering worry.

You are busy listening to the buzzing thoughts in your head, waiting for your next anxiety attack, assessing the threat level, analyzing the next socially acceptable thing to say, and calculating how much longer you can fake your enjoyment before you make your well-rehearsed excuse to run away.

This is what it means to exist in a trauma body. This is life with PTSD, every single day. It's missing the entirety of your life, even while being immersed in beautiful moments with kind friends. Trauma takes you out of the present in the moment, and it doesn't allow you to see what's safe and beautiful right next to you.

FEAR SPOONED ME

Fear spooned my back and stayed.

It cloaked me from behind, spreading itself over
my head and wrapping itself in front of my face.

Fear washed my trust away, leaving stuckness
and worry as my best friends.

Fear pressed my shoulders and cemented my head down,
forcing my eyes to look only at the ground.

It thrust my arms to hang heavily down, my fingers numb,
and it locked all the doors that I wanted to open shut.

Fear's cold breath behind my ear reminded
me that I wasn't welcome here.

Fear spooned me.

It stuck to my legs, forcing me to walk the opposite way,
and it shadowed me with every single step.

Fear spooned me.

At night, its fingers reached into my mind,
penetrating my thoughts from behind,
crippling me with dread running up and down my spine.

Fear kept me awake,
it knew how to keep me deprived.

And though it's never left my side,
it tells me that it's only just arrived.

SCARED

MY NEED TO CONTROL YOUR EMOTIONS, BEHAVIOR, and choices, came from my deep fear of being unsafe. It came from my uncertainty about what could happen to me next. My tower of uncertainty is a powerless place to be, even if from the outside, it looks like the self-exalting behavior of an authoritarian despot.

SHAME

Shame, shame, here you are.

Of course, you're never gone long enough to make
me believe you've completely disappeared.

But why come back tonight?

I don't want to diminish my own light, to
silence my voice, to make myself small.

I need to be a competent adult.

Chew me up and spit me to the curb, I know the drill.

I will recover, I know that by now, so let's just get on with it.

It's not the first time.

I need to be a competent adult
tonight, not a wounded child.

Not tonight.

SELF-RETALIATION

RETALIATING AGAINST MYSELF WAS A BETTER response than allowing others to keep retaliating against me. It was a way to maintain some crumb of dignity. Between them punishing me or me punishing myself, I chose to punish myself, and no one was a worse enemy than I was to me.

Self-alienation, self-hatred, self-discipline, self-demand, self-criticism, and self-destruction—all the wars I lived through, this self-imposed war against myself was the most difficult. But I stayed put, and I kept my dignity. I retained a sense of control over myself and, with it, a sense of integrity.

It was a coping and survival mechanism that allowed me to believe I still had a choice for myself and my own agency. Even if I was self-retaliating, at least it was done to me, by me. It was my decision. That is the core of abuse and trauma.

RESIGNING

The following is dedicated to my fifteen-year-old self, and to all the children of the former Yugoslavia, as well as every child who has been affected by war and displacement who experienced the emptiness of Resignation Syndrome.

CONTENT WARNING: THIS ESSAY MENTIONS SUICIDE.

GIVING UP IS A PLACE WHERE HELPLESSNESS AND hopelessness collide. It's a state where a heavy sense of powerlessness and exhaustion converge upon you. From there you go one step further, into a state where you resign.

Being in a resigned state is more difficult than thinking about ending your life, or even trying to end your life. Thinking about suicide requires some level of mental and physical work. Not only do you need to think about how to do it, but you also need to have some level of energy to follow through.

Resignation means there is no life energy left in you. It's a place where you don't care how much longer you will live in pain. You can't eat, drink, walk or talk. It's a place of deep mental, spiritual, and physical nothingness. This is called Resignation Syndrome. It's a place of complete catatonic shutdown. It's a place where you don't have the energy to die, and also, where you don't have the energy to live.

HOW IT FEELS TO HAVE TRAUMA AND PTSD

AS SOMEONE WHO HAS LIVED THROUGH AND SUR-vived numerous wars, who—for years—has been in the midst of horrors caused by humans, I would describe PTSD and trauma as a state where everything in your body feels unreliable and unable to support you. Everything in you feels and sounds like terror. It's a state where there is the constant high-velocity impact of being under threat.

The threat is inside of you, it is your body. It's also around you, above you, and below you. It constantly feels—twenty-four seven, for years—like every bullet from every gun in all directions is aimed and coming at you. Every bomb and every grenade is coming down upon you. PTSD is believing there's a minefield below you, in you, around you, and above you. It's an inescapable place of deep loneliness and enduring fear.

All of this threat overloads your nervous system, which can't keep carrying you. All you can do is just hope that you will not explode, like a ticking time bomb, every single day, every single hour, sometimes even minute to minute.

It is important to know that you can have PTSD without living through wars as I have. Any threat constantly coming toward you can trigger PTSD. For me, the threat was never munition, but people. Feeling a constant sense of danger and uncertainty about when, or whether, you are going to be killed, abused, shamed, ridiculed, or mocked, and then be left to deal with it in isolation can cause PTSD.

4

TRAUMA
INSIGHTS

JEALOUSY IS NOT ENVY

DON'T ACCEPT SOMEONE'S JEALOUSY. BEING ON THE receiving end of someone's jealousy is harmful and violates your self-esteem and agency. Jealousy fuels abuse in malignant narcissists and sadists because of their deep sense of inadequacy.

Don't confuse envy with jealousy. Envy doesn't cause harm, jealousy does. Envy can be blunt—your feelings might not be considered, you might be taken for granted—but it won't harm you or crush your integrity. Envy motivates people to make things happen. Jealousy prevents things from happening because it's a source of contempt.

When someone is jealous of you, it prevents you from trusting yourself. It has power over you and it feels abusive. It causes you to question your ability and your reality. It kills your happiness, drive for life, and your confidence to connect with others and reach out to the world.

It's the most poisonous emotion in many families. Often, parents enable one of their children to be abused, cast out, and destroyed by allowing or even encouraging jealousy between siblings.

These parents come to the child they've set on a pedestal, saying things like, "Love your brother and don't show him up! He's not as smart as you," or "You need to help your poor sister; you're better at this than she is." All the while, you received nothing but contemptuous looks from your siblings' jealous eyes.

This kind of treatment causes you to normalize jealousy from your coworkers, friends, in-laws, and others. Out of habit, embarrassment, or shame, you make yourself wrong to allow them to be right. You step into the shadows so they can stand in the light. Envy might ruin your day, but jealousy destroys you for life.

THERE IS NO RUNNING TOWARD

THE TRAUMA AND PTSD MIND WILL NEVER ALLOW YOU to run toward anyone or anything. Before you can run toward someone or something, you first need to have a safe person or space to run toward. In that refuge, that safe haven, you would be able to rest and feel protected. That does not exist in trauma. In trauma, there has never been a safe person or a place you could run to, and that possibility can't even exist in its realm.

The trauma brain lives in a state of always running away from something or someone. The mind and body of trauma are defined by running away from danger and not toward something safe. The trauma mind doesn't trust people. It cannot believe there is a safe person to run toward because that safe people don't exist in the first place. And there is no safe destination to run toward, either.

The trauma mind is always being chased by a desperate hope that you will reach safety by running from shame, isolation, insults, anxiety, mistreatment, pain, poverty, discrimination, wars. You are running from some threat to safety, never toward someone to feel safe. That running away to feel safe comes from a desperate hope that there is a place where only peace and harmony exist. A place of rest, nothing else. It is a place where the push and pull of life ceases and there is only the constant oasis of equilibrium. It is not a place where a specific safe human exists to embrace you and hold you.

The reality is that there isn't a constant safe place. Life is an amalgamation of negative, neutral, and positive experiences, but it is so hard for trauma bodies to get that realization, to live in that space. How could you get there when you need to *run from* in order to survive, all the time, all your life. That is why trauma is so tremendously exhausting.

What you can do is to find peace and safety in micro-moments of your day. You will find them when you are not running from pain, but running toward noticeable safety in your body, environment, and thoughts. Notice one molecule of safety in your body, one pleasant thought in your mind, one tiny beam of light in your room. Harmony and peace can exist in your world when you build and gain access to safety, and when you stop running away from pain.

Harmony and peace are not constant states and never will be. Life is about building resilience so that you can face turmoil when it happens but also move consciously toward safety to rest and have peace.

DO YOU ALLOW IT OR DO YOU COMPLY?

WHEN YOU ALLOW SOMEONE TO BENEFIT FROM YOUR time, body, skills, or personal things, you give them access to your being and what belongs to you. It's your choice, and a gift to whoever you share it with.

There is consent, agreement, and respect. You keep your full autonomy and integrity, which allows you to feel generous. This kind of giving feels right.

Compliance on the other hand, is when you give of yourself, including your body, your time, your belongings, and your skills, to others in order to survive and remain safe. With compliance, you override what you truly want in order to be safe, loved, and belong. There is no consent.

In order not to lose a friend, you might lend your car to them. In order not to lose your boyfriend, you comply with having sex, even though you don't want to.

In order to keep your boss from getting mad, you might overcommit yourself to work, offering an excess of your skills and time, which you are not paid for.

In order to keep the peace in your family, you might not plan a vacation with your friends, and instead spend the holidays with them.

How often in your life have you truly consented to sharing yourself, and how often have you been compliant? That is the difference between a normal life, where you give the gift of yourself to others, and a conditioned life of compliance, given without your true consent.

RAGING FATHERS AND APPEASING MOTHERS

HOW MANY TIMES HAVE YOU CASUALLY SAID, "YES, OF course, I will do that," while feeling constricted and immobile on the inside?

That constriction is stored fear, discomfort, anger, and insecurity. People might think of you as a people-pleaser, or you might recognize that pattern within yourself, but what you need to understand is that your intelligent nervous system is using your social engagement skills to prevent situations from becoming dangerous to you.

If you express anger, or fear, or even say no, things might get worse. That's why you respond with appeasement as a way to stay safe. You become a yes person. You become an enabler of other people's behavior.

You said yes to something you didn't want to do or have the ability to do, but only because your sense of fear was stronger than your sense of your own limitations. Most of the time, you're not aware of those responses. This is simply your bid for survival. It comes quickly with a sense of urgency as response to a threat.

If you were brought up in a family with a raging father and an appeasing mother, most likely you would mirror the same response. Looking back at your childhood, it appeared to you that your mother was enabling your father's rage, and in a way she was. She wasn't able to stop it. It seemed like she was fine with the violence in your home, even compliant with it, implying to you from an early age that rage is something you need to accept and live with.

You might blame your mother for how she didn't protect

her children. In truth, you and your siblings were abandoned by both of your parents. It felt like being betrayed by them, by his explosive wrath and her complacency. It is desolating for a child to grow up in a home like this.

Though your mother's behavior was a betrayal to you, it was also an appeasement response by her nervous system to attempt to manage your father's violence by becoming a people-pleaser. That is how your mother felt safe in the moment, and she believed she was keeping her children safe, too. There is nothing motherly or nurturing in this biological response. Her intent was never to harm you. Appeasing your father was her trauma response, her biology taking over.

Most people with this type of people-pleasing, fawn response tend to deny and minimize what happened. It's hard to get to them to see what is actually happening in the home. They will even defend the abuser's behavior and try to make it seem like it's not so bad. If you are now a parent, you can make a different choice for your children. After experiencing rage or partner-violence, look at your options and make choices that protect your children and break the trauma cycle. This is where you have control. Doing so is challenging. It requires you to have a system of support in place; the maturity, wisdom, education and knowledge of how to safely exit a violent situation; and enough sustainability to survive, but it can happen.

Unfortunately for many of us, we felt betrayed by our parents growing up; we were emotionally abandoned in our homes with our raging fathers and appeasing mothers. Our parents were never able to break the cycle.

CHILDHOOD TRAUMA

NEGLECTED OR INVADED. THERE IS NO IN-BETWEEN for you in the midst of developmental trauma.

I AM CONSTANTLY JUDGING YOU

IS YOUR PARTNER, OR YOUR FRIEND, OR YOUR CHILD, living up to your expectations? Do they perform the way you think they should, the way you think they have to? If they need more time to process, learn, and figure things out, how quickly do you judge them?

How quickly do they irritate you, and how long before you can't tolerate them doing things their own way, even for a second longer? What will happen to you if they don't meet your standards? What will happen if they take time to decide?

Do you feel discomfort, or fear that something might happen to you if the people around you don't deliver their best, as you demand?

The main questions to consider are: who in your childhood was ignorant, unaware, or too slow to step up and protect you? Whose averageness and ignorance caused you harm? Whose inaction, and whose action, took your safety away?

That trauma in you is still alive and demands everyone

around you to be responsive, agile, and to deliver nothing but perfection, all so you can be safe. Others don't see that.

They see you as an adult who's never satisfied with them, no matter what they do for you. They see you as someone whose bar of expectation is unreachable. They see only your next disappointment and demands, and because of this, they will build resentment and hold grudges toward you. They may even leave you. Most likely, you will end up lonely because of these demanding expectations.

Your adult kids will stop visiting you. Your partner will be exhausted by you and no longer see your relationship as a source of love. Your friends will be tired of your constant dissatisfaction with their lives. Who is judging whom? Your encapsulated trauma memory, that scared inner child who was traumatized, is the one judging.

You might not even be aware you're doing it. What you need to do is protect the traumatized parts of your inner child. That scared part of you who seeks constant perfection from others and has such high expectations is afraid of being harmed again. Instead of facing that fear, he or she is making everyone else responsible for your safety.

Why should they be responsible? Why would someone keep doing things for you when it's never enough? As an adult, you are responsible for your safety. It is your job to learn about your limits and rights. You need to educate yourself on your behaviors and how to heal. Fulfilling your demands for perfection so you can keep yourself safe because you experienced trauma is not anyone else's responsibility.

That isn't their burden, and not what they signed up for when they decided to have a relationship with you. Expecting perfection from others so you don't get hurt or retraumatized is a fantasy. In reality, you will end up being abandoned by the people who truly care about you.

SOCIAL ANXIETY

WHEN YOU ARE FACED WITH A PENDING SOCIAL event, all of your body's impulses will urge you to stay home and not go. Home may be lonely, but it's safe.

It's not that you don't have social skills, or that you don't want to have a nice time, but your body viscerally remembers when being in a group of people—whether it was with your family, at work, or at school—made you feel inadequate, ashamed, or humiliated.

The body does indeed keep the score, and now you're an adult, sitting at dinner, while your brain recalls that implicit memory, which literally produces the same physical symptoms as when you were shamed ten or twenty years ago. It recalls that exact moment and causes you to sweat, get flushed, feel immobile, and become hypervigilant, uneasy, and filled with panic, all as a response to that original shame.

That is social anxiety. The nervous system recalls a memory of when you were shamed, insulted, or ridiculed in front of people, and relives that moment every time you're with people again. Essentially, your survival brain still perceives people as a threat rather than a source of safety, and yet you are a social being and have an innate need to explore and connect with the world. You want to take up space. You want to be seen. You want to be heard. You are intelligent and witty. You know so much that you want to share with the world, and yet everything inside of you prevents you from connecting.

Your survival instinct wants you to be safe, regardless of how you long for human connection. It wants to protect you from what it remembers. This is what the inner struggle of social anxiety feels like.

Remember, the people who harmed you don't get the right to deprive you of all the good, genuine, and kind people in the world. Unfortunately, unkind people exist, but there are so many more out there who would not only welcome a connection with you, but will never make you feel ashamed that way again.

SOCIAL ANXIETY POEM

No. Do not pull me down. Enough!
We can't continue to hide.

But, we can also die if we go outside.
We are already dead inside.

No, I cannot stay bent down, confined.
There's no place left to hide.

I can't continue to neither live nor die.

So let's go out, even if we die.

We will take up space, and maybe,
finally make some friends.

I can't watch myself neither live nor die.

So let's go out, we can't stay confined and hide.

Not everyone will do us harm.

We will look for those with kind eyes.

DON'T THINK ABOUT THE FUTURE

WHEN YOU LIVE WITH TRAUMA AND PTSD, THINKING about the future is like adding salt to your wounds. It's like confirming to yourself that you will never have a normal life, that everyone is better than you, and that you will continue to fail.

Thinking about the future with PTSD brings more stuckness and deprivation to your being, and prevents you from recovery. So, don't do it. Don't think about the future, not even what you will do tomorrow, or in two days.

With PTSD, you start recovering by thinking about micro-moments, about tiny tasks that you can accomplish in the next minute, or maybe hour. No one gets to judge you, or say anything to you for this, either. No one is in your skin. Most of the time, we're the ones placing judgment and pressure on ourselves.

If there is someone judging you in your environment, cut them out. Leave them with their ignorance, or better yet, stick them in front of YouTube or have them read about PTSD until they feel ashamed for judging you. Let them read this chapter. Let me lecture them!

When you can't leave your home for days because everything outside is frightening and overwhelming to face, you don't have to. You can turn the knob on your door and sit in front of it. That may be enough for you at that moment. Some days, just going outside on your front porch is a monumental accomplishment.

Take this micro-step. It might look like nothing, but for someone with PTSD it is more than enough. It can feel like a really big step. Moving out of the bed that you don't want to leave just to sit on the porch *is* a big step.

If you feel anguish or guilt because you think you're a burden to your partner or your family, taking the micro-step of saying, "Thank you; can I hold your hand?" is enough.

Reaching out for someone's hand, connecting to the eyes of someone you appreciate, and saying thank you is tremendously difficult for your system because it first needs to move through the states of shame and inadequacy, which is already difficult enough. What looks like a micro-step to others is the equivalent of climbing K2 for someone with PTSD.

Coming out of your bedroom when your family has friends over, and just allowing yourself to approach your favorite person in the group and thank them for coming is huge.

Telling them, "I don't have the ability to socialize yet, but I just wanted to come downstairs and see you," and then going back to your bedroom is genuinely more than enough.

This is where you are, and it's important to respect that. You may only have three minutes with someone, and that's enough for you right now. Looking at your face in the mirror and saying, "I'm here for you," when you're full of bruises and scars, is enough.

Showing up at your support group on Zoom for just ten or fifteen minutes is enough. Deciding to make yourself dinner and feeding yourself while standing on your feet when it feels impossible is enough.

These micro-steps are more than enough, and they are enormous, monumental accomplishments for a PTSD body. Once you complete them, then you can practice repeating these micro-steps every day.

One day you will be able to sit outside of your door and

catch the sunlight on your skin. You will be able to reach for your partner's hand and thank them. You will say, "Hi," to a kind friend. You will look in the mirror and say, "I've got you." You will show up in your support group. You will even make yourself dinner.

In the meantime, don't think about the future in this phase of recovery. You will have plenty of time for that, just not now. Now you are rebuilding your life in small tasks. All those micro-tasks are moving you into your future, where you will regain your abilities and become an even better version of yourself. You will get this, just not right now.

YOUR ENTITLEMENT

YOU ARE ENTITLED TO BE VALUED AS A HUMAN BEING. It's your human right. People don't need to agree with your choices or opinions for you to have value. They can react, but they don't have the right to disrespect or dehumanize you.

You inherently have value. Living in a household filled with trauma, you normalized being devalued. You normalized being talked over, dismissed, mocked, bullied, harassed, assaulted, yelled at, controlled, threatened, shamed, minimized, and intimidated.

You normalized your dehumanization. That's the core of trauma. Maybe it was normal in your home, or in your environment, but this is not what happens in healthy homes. Homes that are filled with trauma normalize dehumanization and devaluation.

You normalized crimes committed against you. You didn't

know that it could be different. You may have been abused by adults when you were a helpless, unprotected child—child who believed the abuse was normal. It was all you knew.

Now as an adult, you need to relearn what is normal.

Consider educating yourself to learn what healthy behavior is, what people are allowed and not allowed to do to you. You learn this through personal psycho-education, support groups, reading books, attending workshops, and going to therapy. Learn what intimidation, harassment, violations, and insults are. They are crimes against your humanity.

Your right, your human right, is to be valued and respected as a person who exists in this world. People don't have to agree with you, but they do not have a right to devalue you.

SHAME NEVER EXPIRES

THE MOMENT YOU EXPERIENCE TRAUMA, SHAME comes alive inside of you. The traumatic experience stops, but not the shame. It never stops. The shame always stays alive and always follows you. It will die with you. This is what trauma does to our innocence and dignity.

WHO DO YOU
NOT SEE?

DEAR READER, YOUR EYES—WHICH ARE LONGING
and searching for approval in others—never look inward at
your beauty and kindness. Genuinely kind people can see
your essence. They aren't searching for a fantasy. They are
seeking an authentic human connection, the same way you
are.

Show up as your true self, without pretense, fluff, or
excessive effort, and see what happens. Good people will
stick with you and the artificial relationships will naturally
fall away, which is a blessing.

You might believe you have nothing of value to offer
unless you provide something to others. The real task is
to provide for yourself first, and not do things for others'
approval, and watch how things change for the better. Provide yourself with what you were longing for from others:
appreciation, acknowledgment, tenderness, time to make
a choice, patience, and acceptance.

Before you can be anything to anyone else, you have to
make yourself your most valuable companion, gain back
your trust in yourself, and be loyal to yourself. As one client
said in a session, "It needs to be from me, for me."

What you'll notice by doing this is how much of your life
force is directed toward your own satisfaction, into your
craft, and into the life you create for yourself.

You will never disappoint yourself, nor your genuine
friends. This is what you will learn, and what matters the
most. From then on, you will be the one approving of others,
not vice versa.

THE HERO YOU
KEEP DISMISSING

IS WHAT YOU'RE FEELING CAUSED BY THE STRESS OF regular life, or abuse? What are you facing now? If you're dealing with challenges at work, with your relationships, with boundaries, with money, with your health, then this is regular life, not abuse. However, your body feels this stress as a tremendous threat, and can produce the same visceral state as when you were abused.

It can feel the same way it did when you were a helpless child, or an adult being hurt and violated. It's important to see the difference between the two. First, remind yourself of what you actually survived, and that you did survive. It happened and it's in the past.

Place a timestamp on that memory and look at the date. It sounds simple, but trauma is all about being stuck in time. The trauma body doesn't know the abuse is over. So look at the calendar. What day and year is it now? Remind yourself that you are an adult now who pays bills and drives a car.

Remind yourself that you are not a child, and that you are not in the abusive space you were before. Also, compare the facts with what you are facing now. Locate the threat. Is it actually a threat, a perpetrator that you are facing, or is it a moody partner, a miserable boss, or an obnoxious neighbor?

There is a big difference. So, locate the threat, if there is any. Keep those two things—time and location—in mind when you get activated. Then, remember where you came from. You came from abuse and trauma. You survived it. Don't underestimate the resiliency and capabilities you gained by surviving neglect and abuse.

Are you even aware of that? Do you recognize what you went through and what you gained in your toolbox to help you with the challenges you now face as an adult? If you survived a lack of support as a child, or even as an adult, then there is an imprinted resiliency in you that helps you survive "regular" life challenges. If you were a survivor of abuse and trauma, then you are not a snowflake. People may think you're fragile, as if you're a porcelain doll who will break at any moment, but you survived the unthinkable.

Next, it's important to do a data check. Ask yourself if this is actually an abuser who is trying to violate your human rights by leaving you without a choice, or if you are dealing with an obnoxious or toxic coworker who you can report to HR, call your lawyer about, or talk with your therapist about? Can you educate yourself on your rights, or ask for a change of department?

Do you actually not have a choice, or are you being reminded of a past in which you didn't have any choice? Are you an adult now, or are you fifteen once again? What is today's date? What is the year? Slowly ask yourself these questions and let your body absorb the answers.

Make a timeline of pictures from the year you were born up to now, to remind yourself of how far you've come. If you don't have photos, take some from the magazines you read when you were that age. Look at how far you've come.

Remind yourself what you've overcome and how much strength is inside of you, even if there is a part of your brain that is dismissing this as you read it. Yes, I know how the trauma brain works because I have one, too. Don't dismiss what you're reading. Let it sink in, and when you have to face the jackasses in your life, remind yourself that they are *just* jackasses, not the predators and perpetrators from your past.

FEAR, DANCE WITH ME

Fear, where have you been? I thought you
went away, for almost a full day.

You want to nest inside of me and make me restless? Sure.

Come, come to me and take over, I know the drill.

Yes, spread yourself out and flood all over me.
Hold my breath, compress my heart, and squeeze my gut.
But this time, you will dance with me.
Yes, this time, we'll just move.

I can feel you all over my spine and across my prickled skin.
I feel you in my throat. I feel you in my trembling voice.

We are like lovers, old and drained, never
giving ourselves a second chance.

Yes, come and suck me up, we know the drill by now.

But this time you will dance with me
as I allow you to take me in.

Move, move, move with me.
Wrap around me, cloak me. I will surrender.
I know the drill, and yet, this time we will move and dance.

This could be fun. I know you so well.
There is nothing new about the two
of us. We are deeply bound.

So let's dance, and wait. Why do you feel
so light? Are you leaving me now?
What's wrong? Don't go, we are finally having fun.
I'm here. I know the drill, wash over me.
You are the partner I know so well. Take me
in. You see how easily I surrender?

I don't want to, said the fear, *I don't need you.*
You look like an adult for the first time.
With you leading, I feel protected.
You found ease and acceptance. You
blossomed with independence.

There is a trustworthy voice I can hear.
You know me, the fear said. *We are old partners,*
but I am so young. It is me, your inner child.

I was pushing you, hurting you, shaking you
so you could stay alive, not dead inside,
not compliant to everyone all the time.
I needed protection from the adult you.
I never meant to be mean to you.

I am leaving you now.
It has been four decades since I let myself rest.
Now, I can because I know I will finally
be in protective hands.

EMOTIONAL ABUSE

MENTAL ABUSE IS INSIDIOUS. IN THE BEGINNING, IT may feel like it's not that big of a deal, nothing major, abrupt, or even definable. There may be no cursing or any verbal insults at all. It happens in tiny, toxic micro-moments. It's like mold. You can't yet see it growing in your home, you can't pinpoint where it started, so you just live with it as your health and well-being deteriorate.

You don't know why you're suffering. You don't even realize that you've somehow lost yourself—your old self, who you used to be. Your self-esteem has plummeted and you question yourself about everything. You don't trust your experiences. You feel social anxiety, and somehow you've become invisible and isolated, maybe even scared. It's as if you lost your essence, as if you ceased to exist.

And yet, no harsh words were spoken to you. You didn't witness any rage, or experience any physical violence, but your body still feels like it's been covered with mold. Your body knows something is wrong. Someone has distorted your reality.

The mold is the person you spend time with or live with who is mentally abusing you. Even if you can't put your finger on it, you need to move yourself to a new home, with no trace of mold in it. You deserve a healthy and safe home, free from insidious abuse.

TRAUMA STATE

I am not living, and I am also not dead.

SUICIDE

WHEN A PARENT DIES BY SUICIDE, THEIR CHILD IS left to live their life with deep anger and disgust toward that parent. The anger and disgust hides the deep desperation and betrayal the child feels. The wounded child screams in fear because their parent is no longer there to protect them. They are left in a world where that source of protection is suddenly gone, leaving them unprotected and abandoned.

It instills a deep sense of inner unworthiness in the child. They believe that if they were at all worthy, their parent wouldn't have left them unprotected and alone in the world. When a partner dies by suicide, the surviving partner is left in the same state. This is betrayal trauma.

The child can't yet understand that suicide happens because of two things that happen in the human body. The first is that the person is so tired of their pain and feels unable to endure it any longer. The roles people play in the outside world in order to hide what is happening in their inner world keep them even more isolated in their pain, and this makes them tremendously exhausted.

The second is that the human psyche has a deep love for the rest of the body and wants to help stop the pain by deciding to end their life. That part sees death as the end of suffering, and an opportunity to finally find peace. As a therapist and a trauma survivor, I have so much love and respect for both of these parts.

When society forces everyone to follow an unattainable fantasy and places ever-increasing expectations of heroic-level achievements, then people are bound to feel overburdened and like failures. Living becomes a place of trying not to fail, all to avoid being shamed or judged by society.

Humans are not Hollywood productions. They are frail and strong, and all that exists in between these two extremes. A human is someone with thousands of roles, they should not be forced to maintain only one by a demanding society that crushes their spirit with shame until they die by suicide.

CAN YOU FEEL JOY AND PLEASURE?

DO YOU WONDER WHY YOU CANNOT EXPERIENCE more joy, more pleasure, or more excitement? Do you wonder why—when you start to experience any of it—you feel the instinct to run away and dismiss it from your body as quickly as you can?

It's almost as if it's insulting to your body to feel good.

If you have been shamed or humiliated, your body stays in a state of inhibition. Shame slows you down and makes you almost frozen, paralyzed from feeling joy.

Imagine the amount of shame that is stored in your body if you had to live with someone who continuously shamed or mocked you in front of others? Or perhaps you were humiliated at school when you just wanted to express your playfulness and exuberance? How many times were you shut down in your family, as if you had committed a crime, when you just wanted to dance and exude your life force?

The trauma brain remembers when you were in an expansive, joyful state just before you were humiliated or ridiculed, and your brain doesn't want to ever allow that state again. It's too dangerous, and your brain simply wants to protect you, even now when you live a safe life away from all the bullies.

All of those experiences have a tremendous effect on your nervous system, and those micro-traumas produce so much shame — shame in feeling pleasure, joy, playfulness, goofiness, fun, or even healthy, protective anger. Shame creates the inhibitory state, making you withdraw from others.

You will, as a protective response, resist natural experiences like laughter, joy, expressive movement, humming, singing, playful sex, even anger. You will subconsciously cut down on all of your potentially expansive states, so you never have to experience shame again.

Shame inhibits you. It compresses the possibility of feeling joyful, happy, expansive, and bold. If — God forbid — you do feel it coming up, it will quickly be shut down. This is what shame and humiliation do to us.

LIFE OXYMORON

People harm you. People heal you.

SCHOOLYARD BULLIES

SCHOOL FOLLOWS YOU ALL YOUR LIFE. WHEN YOU ARE rejected by a partner, from a work project, or not invited to be part of a venture opportunity or business deal, it feels like being stabbed in your core and a total dismissal of your value. Your insecurities from school are alive and present again.

It feels like you've lost your identity, and all the therapy, retreats, masterclasses, workshops, and groups — the entire life you built — suddenly vanish and you are left with the old familiar taste of being excluded. A taste you learned in school, where you were othered by friends or by a clique, or when you were picked on and laughed at by a couple of schoolyard bullies.

You didn't know why they chose you, but they did and it felt terrible. Those cruel bullies are still residing inside your trauma mind, as loud, arrogant, and condescending as they were decades ago, the moment you were rejected from the group or told no.

Now, as an adult, you were likely rejected because the project wasn't good enough, the money fell through, or the timing wasn't right. It had nothing to do with you, your identity, or your core values, but those schoolyard bullies left an imprint of unworthiness inside of you.

Most likely, those bullies are good people now, dealing with their own lives, mortgages, and kids, and whoever continued being a bully was probably cast out by adults who can wisely pick their inner circle of friends. So, who cares about them? Let the bullies be bullies. They will never be welcomed in your circle anyway.

When you notice rejection in your current life and it throws you off, remind yourself that it is not coming from those obnoxious kids who hurt you. Hold the wounded child inside of you with your adult self, take them to a nice bookstore or a restaurant, and protect them from all those bullies who caused them pain.

Love your inner child more now than ever. Show them what an awesome adult you have become and how you can deal with life's pitfalls without feeling othered and devastated.

WERE YOU ALLOWED TO SAY "I DON'T KNOW"?

SAYING "I DON'T KNOW" OR "I CAN'T DECIDE RIGHT now" was never an option for the trauma survivor. It's a privilege to not have to make a choice, or be asked to answer in the moment, and to be able to reply, "I will get back to you once I decide."

It's something that's not even possible to think of in the midst of trauma. Once your body moves into a safe space where you can pause, reassess, and be able to figure things out without urgency, it can feel like you won an Oscar. What a privilege! To say, "I don't know, I will get back to you," and remain unharmed!

The survival brain, activated by the nervous system in trauma, doesn't have the luxury of reacting with, "Let's pause. I need to reassess my needs, and if I am not sure, I will get back to you in a day or two." No, it can't imagine such a thing!

The survival brain only functions on urgency and vigilance. Every single second you need to know how to react, what to do, and what to say, so you don't face more harm and pain. That is the trauma brain.

This is why if you see someone quickly respond, or demand an answer immediately, I guarantee it was primed by living in unpredictability and a lack of safety.

Allow yourself to notice this new safe space, one where you can say, "Let me get back to you," or "I don't know."

Bask in it. What a pleasure to know you won't be harmed, shamed, or damaged again. Notice it, use it, and wrap yourself in this privilege. It means you are safe now.

Also, it's important to honor other people's choice to say, "I will get back to you."

Their uncertainty in the moment, and their need to take time to answer you will not harm you, either. You don't need to receive an immediate answer from others to feel safe.

You survived. Bask in the pleasure of this knowledge and of not having to decide or know everything all the time, every hour, every second. Let your heart take a breath and soften back.

WHO KILLED YOUR PLAYFULNESS?

TO BE PLAYFUL AND SILLY MEANS TO FEEL SAFE WITH those around you. I stopped being playful and silly when the people around me became a source of judgment, contempt, and part of the cancel-culture. They killed my playfulness. Games suddenly went from being a source of excitement and connectivity to being a potential for embarrassment and shame.

As an adult, office games or group games of any sort became a stressor; I worried if I would make a fool of myself, and if the heat of shame would redden my face. Anxiety would flood my body at the possibility of being othered. Games could no longer evoke any sense of excitement or fun within me. Being playful meant I would probably end up ashamed.

Who killed your playfulness and silliness? Who deprived you of your innate need to play? We are al born with the need to play, to be curious and to have fun. Just look at animals; their playfulness is an innate instinct.

Unfortunately, humans can deprive each other of the need to be playful. Humans can kill another's excitement, innocence, ease, and fun.

Pay attention to the kids at the playground, and notice who's not a part of the group; who's sitting on the side or anxiously fidgeting when it's time for group play? Who's not in the group when it's play time?

The same applies in your office. Do you love team-building games? If not, read this page one more time, and then track down when your playfulness disappeared? Who killed it?

Who killed your genuine, playful connection with others and moved you into a space of scared self-consciousness and inhibition? Who destroyed your need to be playful, to connect with your friends and other safe people around you?

DISSOCIATION, THANK YOU

AWARENESS OF ABUSE OR TRAUMA IS DANGEROUS. You don't want to be in awareness mode. Imagine the pain you would feel and the impact of what happened to you if you were fully aware of it? So, thank your body for dissociation. Thank your nervous system and your survival brain for guiding you to a numb, floating, dissociative state.

In that space, pain wasn't so painful. There, you could be absent. There, you couldn't fully see your injuries while they were happening. There, you felt less. Dissociation, thank you for protecting me.

RECEIVING EYES

Who received you with their eyes?

Whose words were spoken though soft gazes,
timeless holding, and vast acceptance.

Who held you with their kind eyes?

Who watched over you with their receiving
eyes when the pain was too much?

Who held you with receiving eyes when
your body was crying out?

Who?

No one.

COMPLIMENTS YOU CANNOT RECEIVE

NOTICE HOW QUICKLY YOU DISMISS COMPLIMENTS from others. Notice how quickly you deny even the thought of a micro-niceness about yourself, or any tiny acknowledgment from others. Notice that.

You behave as if there's no possibility in the world that someone else could see goodness in you, because you can't even acknowledge or appreciate your own goodness.

Notice the awkwardness on your face the moment you receive a compliment, and how quickly you brush it off and look away. Notice how you feel compelled to instantly move yourself away from it.

How quickly do you override the compliment with your inner thoughts? *Ah, if only you knew*, you think, *Let me show you my list of failures and inadequacies.* Then, maybe, you change the subject.

Notice those quick overriding thoughts and impulses. That is trauma conditioning, and it is what neglect and abuse does to our souls. You learn to dismiss niceness and goodness about yourself, so you don't become the target of ridicule, shame, or get picked on by your abuser. You learn to dismiss all your good qualities and stay invisible. You learn to hide so you are not a target. Being seen was harmful and costly.

It's a learned trauma response. Dismissal of any worthiness is learned. If you were worthy, big, loud, and proud, how would that have been received in the environment where you grew up or when you lived with someone who wanted to tame your wild heart and soul?

If someone who can harm you hears how good, nice, and

smart you are, it means jealousy and contempt are coming your way. You know you will be punished. Receiving compliments doesn't go well for you.

When you brush off compliments now, as an adult, you are also dismissing the fact that there are genuinely kind and honest people in this world, even if there were not any around when you were conditioned to this response. So, notice your instinct to override and allow yourself to receive a compliment, just for five or ten seconds, if you can.

Allow yourself to receive the compliment and notice that you aren't instantly shamed or embarrassed by someone because of it. The next time, allow that compliment to sink in for a minute or two, or even five. Then, allow it to be with you for a whole day. Let it sink into your body.

Wrap yourself in that compliment and recognize that there are good people in the world, and not everyone is like the person who hurt you. Allow yourself to receive that compliment. You deserve it.

DO YOU LIKE CHANGE?

A PERSON WITH LIVED TRAUMA CAN'T SEE ANY LEVEL of change as something positive. Even going on vacation isn't a positive change, but rather a threat to the structures their system has put in place to keep their body safe from further trauma. A slight change can disrupt the hard-managed routine they've built to perceive and sustain a sense of safety inside of themselves. That is the nature of trauma.

A miniscule change can be triggering and shame-provoking for a trauma survivor. I found myself in the Caribbean sun, deeply ashamed of feeling anxious and unsafe, while everyone around me was dancing and enjoying themselves. I kept questioning and judging myself for how incapable and ungrateful I was for not being able to enjoy my vacation. I shamed myself.

Now, I understand that my trauma response wanted to protect me, even the judgmental part that shamed me. The trauma body and the trauma mind don't respond well to change. They will always fight it.

PAUSE

In urgency, you survive.

In a pregnant pause, you heal.

THE PAIN OF ABANDONMENT

I will give you my will.

I will give you my strength.

I will give you my hope.

I will give you my love.

I will give you my drive.

I will pursue you, telling you how to change
and how you could improve.

I will insist that you should pay attention
and finally make a change.

I will complain.

I will call *you* the problem!

I will yell!

I will blame and point out your mistakes!

I will numb out, zone out, and shout you out.

I will refuse to talk. I'll go to my shell and withdraw.

I will resign.

And I will repeat the same cycle a hundred times,
running from screaming panic so as not to feel rejected,
let down, dismissed and being helpless.

I will abandon myself so as not to
witness others abandoning me.

I will risk my heart.

I will twist my mind.

I will mold my skin.

I will adapt my core.

I will bend my bones.

My desperate heart will cling to the illusion
of will, strength, hope, love, and drive

somewhere in your eyes, so I can lie to
myself and say that I safely belong.

All before another vicious cycle swirls me in an
endless fight to find safety and feel beloved.

WERE YOU CRYING IT OUT?

TRAUMA ALWAYS COMES WITH A TREMENDOUS amount of terror and danger, and crying is a way to help release some of the impact of that trauma from the body. Naturally, the body will move to release it. If you look at animals after they experience the initial shock of an attack, they will roar, shake, and move their body in big, deliberate gestures to release the build-up of trauma.

With people who are living with trauma, just as the enormous fear is building and preparing to be released through crying or screaming, there is another force simultaneously suppressing the tears back into the body. In abuse, openly crying could mean even more punishment or humiliation. To survive, you needed to suppress your tears.

Also, cultural conditioning often labels crying as inappropriate. You might learn from your parents or your community to "hold yourself together" and "not make a fool of yourself" by being "hysterical."

Imagine a battle of natural forces in your nervous system. One force wants to be released naturally by crying out, screaming and shouting, while the other suppresses this survival energy, due to the fear of punishment or how society will see you.

This freezes your nervous system by withholding your survival energy. This suppression is also a source of many illnesses. An enormous amount of survival energy gets stuck in your muscles, organs, digestive system, and nervous system, becoming a ticking time bomb because the body knows it's not safe to release it.

You might even recognize that others are withholding their emotions by looking at their posture. They have a braced, heavy, dense demeanor or a slouched, floppy posture that is reflective of a body that is still holding trauma. In somatic therapy, we call this a trauma body.

When there's an impact on your being and you want to cry, then cry it out and let it go. Allow yourself to wail, scream, and shake. Let it all out and help others do the same. It does not calm them down when you tell them, "Shhh," or "Don't cry," especially when there is initial shock trauma trying to move through their body.

These so-called helpers are actually creating stored trauma in the body of the person who's crying by trying to calm them down, even if their intent is to be helpful.

TRAUMA BOND
WITH MYSELF

YOU CAN LEAVE YOUR FAMILY OF ORIGIN, A HARMFUL sibling, or an abusive partner. You can break all those bonds, and still have a trauma bond with yourself. This is the turmoil of constant rumination inside of you. You will have constant dialogues about what you should say, how you should act, and how you should stand up for yourself.

You continuously seek justice to ease your pain. You seek justice in your head. The cycle of hope, agreement, determination, and harming thoughts or behaviors toward yourself is constant. These are the leftovers. This is life with trauma and PTSD.

Even when you break a trauma bond with the people who hurt you, even if you're not in the same household, or a war zone, or the country where you were ostracized, there is still a trauma bond left inside of you. It will not emigrate elsewhere. It might take a vacation on good days, and be quiet for a moment, but it will always live in the hurt self, in the trauma body.

What you need to keep in mind is that no one gets to decide, judge, or tell you how you should move on, or how — by now — you should be healed. They don't live in a trauma body, and probably know very little about trauma. You do. You own your process, your life story, and the time needed to heal. The complexity of what you live with can't be seen from the outside. Don't let anyone make you feel inadequate about your recovery journey and how long it lasts.

WHAT IS THE RIGHT THERAPY?

THE RIGHT THERAPY IS ABOUT ALLOWING YOURSELF to recognize and express your needs while receiving help and safe support. The right therapy is about becoming aware that you are an independent adult.

It is about your body recognizing it can soften into the safety of being nurtured by the protection, care, and support of others, and trust the capabilities of your body. This is what the right therapy feels like.

WHY ARE YOU SO RIGID AND SELF-RELIANT?

HOW TIGHTLY ARE YOU HOLDING ONTO THE STRUCtures you—and only you—built around yourself? How tightly are you holding onto your plans, protocols, and their execution? How rigid are you?

Can you allow yourself to change your plans and opinions? Can you pivot, readjust, change your mind, or call someone for help? Is there any wiggle room in your mind for how you'll execute your plans? Or is it a rigid, inflexible procedure you need to stick to, no matter what?

Is allowing someone to help or steer the wheel—instead of you—even an option? Can someone take your place and take over? Would you feel relief, or a sense of disruption and unease? This clinging to the structure you built around your life, of your plans, of your way, is the only way your system feels safe.

The reason you are so rigid and self-reliant is that you learned from a young age that you couldn't trust or lean on others. That comes from a history of betrayal trauma.

The trauma brain is certain that if you let go of your plans, no one will help you, no one will embrace you, and no one will keep you safe and supported when you fall down and fail. There is no one. Your brain remembers that it doesn't have any support because it never did in the past. It remembers how, when you were growing up, there was no one in life to truly lean on.

You learned to cling to the life you built with the tips of your fingers, all by yourself. Your grip is tenuous at best.

Because of this, you stick to your plans in solitude, just so you never have to go back to that pit of loneliness and pain. That is why failing is never an option, and why you stick so rigidly to the execution of your plans.

Keep in mind that healing begins when we allow ourselves to trust in people again. We need to learn to trust others. It doesn't have to be many people, but at least a few. We heal when we can lean into our support system, and into the safe hands of others. We heal when we don't feel as isolated and lonely as we did our entire lives, and then our rigidness and self-reliance will ease, and the flow of spontaneity will arrive.

CLINGING WITH THE
TIPS OF MY FINGERS

I constricted and braced, tightly holding all of my weight.

I clung to the walls I built with my two hands.

I knew if I let go, no one would be there to catch me.

I would fall into an empty pit, filled with old misery.

It would be the same place I promised
myself I would never return.

There were no hands to hold me in
that familiar abyss of despair.

That pit reminded me that there was no
one to caress me or lift me up.

I learned to armor and constrict myself in order to survive.

Failing was never an option in my mind.

Neither was changing my mind.

UNCERTAINTY

UNCERTAINTY IS THE BIGGEST TRIGGER FOR TRAUMA survivors. It moves all the stored munitions of our trauma and explodes through us as rumination on critical thoughts, self-judgment, overcontrolling, manipulation, over-preparing, sweating, anxiety, over-clinging, and overeating.

It even overrides our current age. We get transported to the age of our trauma. We might go back to the age of seven, or twelve, or twenty-two.

Uncertainty also creates a place of overwhelm and unnerving hypervigilance in our bodies and minds. One of the ways to move yourself out of this state is to name things that are certain in that moment.

Those certainties can be as simple as reminding yourself that your door is locked, that your TV show is waiting for you, that your dog needs a walk, that the bill on your table needs to be paid, that your children need to get to practice, that you can take a bath, that you can call your friend or see your therapist, that you are forty-five years old and not sixteen, that today is this date and not the date when the trauma happened.

Focus on whatever it is that is certain in your life right now, like the routine of your day. Routine is something you can control, adjust, and change. Notice the things around you, and let your body become aware of them. Let your body, eyes, mind, and energy absorb the things at this moment that are certain.

Don't forget to breathe in. Inhale and renew the certainty of your routine, the facts and data of your space, and exhale to release the uncertainty. Repeat, and allow your eyes to land on three certain things in your space, perhaps a chair, a plant, and a painting. Inhale and renew your certainty in this moment, and then repeat again.

THE RICHNESS PEOPLE CANNOT SEE IN YOU

YOU COULDN'T ALLOW ANYONE TO SEE JOY IN YOUR eyes. You learned to vacate your excitement well. Any joy would be taken away. Your abuser wanted to see you hurt. You were never allowed to express that hurt, either. Your abuser would feed off of it. So you learned to numb yourself and shut down from the outside.

You kept a flat affect, allowed no muscle movements, no raising of your hands in a joyful impulse to express happiness. You didn't allow any expressions, especially not in your eyes. The safest way for you to survive was to not show anything on the outside. You learned to hide so well.

Yet, what was — and still is — inside of you is a realm of the most vast intelligence and expressions, filled with all kinds of imagination, fifth dimensions, ideas, dreams, wishes, angels, fairies, guides, allies, and superheroes. It's a universe of harmony, exploration, humanness, and it holds the doors of magic.

This is a world you built in order to escape. There, you were beloved by the king and queen, and you found a palace inside where you could be anything you wanted — especially free. All of that wonder would be punished if it was seen on your face, if it rose to the surface of your skin.

Here, with all your imagined friends, you could fly, explore, and laugh. Everyone belonged in your magical world. Your essence was untouched. You could be exactly who you are.

One beautiful side effect of this imagined world is the creativity it unleashed in your mind. When you express that creativity through writing, music, or any other medium, it will leave people who get it in awe.

That magic can't be felt or understood by others. Who cares? The people who have still, expressionless faces on the outside, and a rich, magical world on the inside, will celebrate you, cry with you, cheer for you, look up to you, and hold you as you are. These are your earth angels.

So, let your richness be expressed. It will be received by people who built the same intricate worlds for the same reasons you did. Let yourself fly. Let your face finally express the bliss you learned so well to hide.

HOW DO I HEAL?

HEALING IS WHAT SURVIVAL TAUGHT YOU NOT TO DO. Survival taught you to stay silent because speaking up would cause you more harm. Healing only happens when you are able to share your story, your thoughts, and your experiences. Survival taught you to not take up space and, instead, to hide.

Healing means being seen amongst others and looking into kind eyes that hold you with respect. Survival is trusting no one and being self-reliant. Healing is learning to lean into others and trust them. It is being able to surrender, to even one person, and opening yourself up to receiving support.

Survival is judging and criticizing yourself until you achieve unattainable perfection. Healing is allowing yourself to stumble, and recognizing you will be supported, not shamed or ridiculed because you made a mistake.

Survival is getting stuck and frozen until the danger passes. Healing is allowing your body to move again, and to move, dance, walk, and run with it. No one shows as much bravery and courage as the person on a journey to heal themselves from trauma. I salute you. Be as kind to yourself as you are brave.

5

SELF ADVOCACY
AND TRUTH IN
CYNICISMS

I'M PAYING YOU, YET I'M SORRY I'M INCONVENIENCING YOU

ASKING FOR A SERVICE THAT YOU ARE PAYING FOR CAN reenact the neglect you experienced growing up. That feeling you have now as an adult is the exact feeling you had when you asked your mother or father to do something for you. Maybe it was when you needed them to buy you shoes, or drive you somewhere, or some other simple thing, and you saw frustration or annoyance in their eyes when you asked.

They made you feel as if they had to go through the trenches of war to do something for you. It was as if your request was an enormous burden, an annoyance, and an inconvenience in their oh-so-busy lives. You mirrored this as you grew up, believing that asking anyone for anything will upset and annoy them.

The outcome of that upbringing was that you felt rejected, unworthy, embarrassed and ashamed for just asking. Now as an adult, how would it feel to ask for a favor from a friend or coworker? Can you do it casually and effortlessly, without a second thought, or is it a dreadful thing to even imagine?

That is why adult children of neglectful parents never ask for anything. You would be hard-pressed to find one trauma survivor who isn't self-reliant, or who had to be growing up. You learned to stop asking others, and this imprint of rejection and unease follows you, even when you are paying hundreds of dollars for a service, and even if you are the head of a corporation. It never leaves you. The embarrassment of asking for your needs to be met brings so much unease into your body.

You are an adult. You make money, you might run your own business or have a team working for you, and yet when you pay for any service — like getting a haircut, having your house cleaned, repairing a leak in your office, or maintaining your car—you might feel intensely uneasy and filled with dread just having to ask for it.

You feel as though you're imposing, even though you're paying them for their expertise, which is how they make a living. Because expressing your wants can be a nerve-racking prospect, you might experience embarrassment if you have to ask for any corrections or adjustments to the work that they did, or to their bill. It's possible that you'll just stop talking and nod your head in agreement. It's possible that you'll always settle for less, even if you know you deserve better.

You don't want to be in their way, and you feel like you can only be thankful, never openly upset, even if you receive shitty service. The abuse you experienced makes you tolerate lower standards, even when you're paying for it.

Don't let it happen. Don't let people take advantage of you. Let them feel uncomfortable, let them be cornered, not you. Expect fair treatment and quality service; expect what you've paid for.

WHEN IS MY TIME COMING?

I haven't even started living and I am already too old.
Who are those younger people around me,
working, living their lives, taking up space, and
following their dreams and wishes?
Isn't that supposed to be me, finally?

When is my time coming?

New generations are taking up space I never took.
But what about me?
My entire life, I was cautious of my elders,
obediently waiting for my turn and
their permission to start living.
Now, seeing my older self, I am almost
embarrassed and apologetic
toward younger crowds when I want to take up space.
It feels like I am stealing something from them
and that I need to hide, and let them live.

Is my time ever coming?

INSTANT DYING

ALL THAT YOU HAVE LEARNED IN THE THERAPIES, workshops, courses, self-help books, and retreats; all the psychoeducation you've done and degrees you earned, vanish in a second when even a small health concern arises. A strange headache, or a pain below your ribs, can send you into a deep trauma state in a matter of seconds.

This is exactly what trauma does to your life. It destroys your trust that you are capable of overcoming challenges, even though you overcame unspeakable hardships, and the onset of an unknown ache can instantly retraumatize you.

How is it that small things like this can set you off in a tailspin, where you believe death is the only outcome? Why is it that you lose all knowledge and trust in yourself?

It's not the outcome of death that scares you. What scares you is your expectation of powerlessness and loneliness encompassing you, while you simultaneously move toward the possibility of dying.

Living with abuse and neglect causes you to continuously feel powerless and lonely, as if you're actively dying, not living. That's exactly where the survival mind goes when it feels pain in your body. It tells you that you will die, but the traumatizing part is that it also tells you that no one will be there for you, and so you hide in your powerlessness and loneliness.

You are convinced that no one will be there for you, or that people will run away from you because you're a burden. You also have no trust that your body will be able to recover. You're convinced that your body will betray you, or that it doesn't have the capacity to overcome being sick. Yet, that same body overcame a ridiculous amount of turmoil and is fully capable of healing.

Your wonderful trauma body never left or betrayed you. You are holding this book and reading it or listening to this book being read. That is what your body is doing right now, holding and reading, or listening.

Your body is with you all the time. Trust your body and your mind will follow. You have handled way more than being sick. You can trust that resilience inside of you.

I AM A CHEAP ARTIST

I am a cheap artist of fake expressions,
hiding behind deep depression.

I am excited, I am passionate, I am happy, I am delighted.

I am a cheap artist of fake expressions,
hiding behind deep depression.

I am proud, I am helpful, I am content, I
am amazed, I am inspired.

I am a cheap artist of fake expressions,
hiding behind deep depression.

I am nonchalant, I am buoyant, I am
relaxed, I am easygoing, I am casual.

I am a cheap artist of fake expressions,
hiding behind deep depression.

I am mindful, I am grounded, I am composed,
I am collected, I am awakened.

I am a cheap artist of fake expressions,
hiding behind deep depression.

I am a leader, I am quick, I am intelligent.
I am a driver, I am competent, I am agile, I am an achiever.
I am a trailblazer, I am a doer!

I am a cheap artist of fake expressions,
hiding behind deep depression.

I am kid-friendly, pet-friendly, community-
friendly, team-friendly, parent-friendly,
partner-friendly, environmentally-friendly, BIPOC-
friendly, LGBTQIA and 2S+-friendly!

I am a cheap artist of fake expressions,
hiding behind deep depression.

I am growing, I am reflecting, I am contemplating, I
am personally developing, I am vibrating on the right
frequency, I am envisioning, I am manifesting!

I am a cheap artist of fake expressions,
hiding behind deep depression.

YIELDING

DO YOU YIELD FOR EVERYONE ELSE'S CONVENIENCE? Have you spent your life in the back of the room, being well-mannered, waiting for your turn to speak, smiling, waiting to be invited, waiting to be included, and waiting to share your opinion? Have you spent your life waiting on the outskirts and yielding to others?

I let everyone go first, instead of me. I let others speak, state their opinions, and show their wit. I let others share their experiences, their travel stories, their manifestation boards, their thrills about mastermind groups and more.

I yielded to others. I let them talk. I listened and let them be the center of attention—all the time—while politely waiting for my turn. I let their choices and opportunities always come first. I believed they were somehow more special, more beautiful, and certainly more competent than me. I was convinced they were better. I told myself:

Don't inconvenience them! Don't say anything! They might get bored or offended. Let them shine! Yield to them! They have more of a right to take up space! They deserve it, not you. They know more than you do. They even look better.

Yield to them! Let them smile! Let them shine! Stay quiet in the corner! Press your spine into the wall, stay silent and small! Keep that smile on your face, stay well-mannered, even as your life is passing you by. That hope that they will notice you and yield for a moment will never be fulfilled. So, stay quiet and keep pretending you are still engaged.

The reality is that your turn is never coming. You will never receive the permission or even the consideration you are waiting for. That helplessness is learned through trauma. You need to learn that you have the right to take space and claim your turn by asserting yourself.

You need to speak up, claim your space, and when someone stops you or overrides you, push back and do the same until they yield to you and let you talk and shine, as you did all those years for them. You don't wait for your turn anymore. You make your turn happen.

YOU ARE NOT CURSED

THE TRAUMATIZED MIND NEEDS TO CREATE MEANING. It needs to explain why the abuse and trauma happened. In our despair, we might believe we have been cursed, or that we have inherited some curse from our ancestors or from our past lives and we are paying for it in this lifetime.

This is not the case. What you experienced was not the result of a curse; it happened because you had a bad person in your family, or you encountered a bad person, who harmed you. A bad person can be someone who is ignorant and sick, or mean and sick. Both are harmful. The second group intends to harm, while the first group does so unintentionally and out of pure ignorance.

The second group is psychopathic. Acknowledging that someone in your family has psychopathic behavior can feel very disruptive, almost offensive. It is unsettling and scary because you might be breaking family loyalty by even think-ing about it.

But what are you actually breaking? You're breaking loy-alty to the douchebag in your family, loyalty to a narcissist, loyalty to a bully, loyalty to an abuser. Just look at the data; how many people in the world are psychopaths? One in two hundred people in Europe, and one in one hundred in the U.S.

These psychopaths do not live in some far-off land behind seven mountains and over seven rivers. No, that psy-chopath can be your next-door neighbor, your boss, your coworker, your father, your sister, or your partner.

What you experienced was not a curse. It was your being in the presence of a sick person who continuously harmed you, and your family's loyalty gave them a free pass. Did your mother whisper in fear for you to not tell anyone what hap-pened? Did she minimize it, or were you threatened by your father to remember what happens in the family stays in the family? How convenient for the abuser!

It's not a curse and it's not karma. It was your being placed in proximity to psychopaths.

UNLESS YOU DO

IN TRAUMA, YOU INHERENTLY BELIEVE YOU'RE A burden to others. You're convinced that with any interaction, you will be perceived as too much, as a nuisance of some sort, unless you make yourself so smart, so informed, such an expert, someone who is always on top of things, always available, always of service, and always diligent—for others.

You're an inconvenience unless you make yourself into the perfect package for others to consume. Only then might you not be a burden to your friends, partners, family, and coworkers. Only then might you belong, or even exist! Only then might you be allowed to be in the presence of others.

In the trauma mind, it's hard to believe in the possibility that someone in your life—whether that be someone in your office, in your social circles, at the gym, or even your partner—genuinely wants to be with you. You! And not for what you do, but for who you are. You can't believe that they just want to be in your presence, that they just want to sit with you and enjoy the day.

This feeling of being a burden is an embodied state. It always follows you. It's constantly there. The way you try to get rid of it is through perfectionism, by adopting ridiculously high expectations of yourself, being overly responsible for others, and by constantly doing for and serving others. There's always the next thing you have to do. And God forbid you ask for help and someone actually goes out of their way for you.

Take a moment here. Notice how hard it is for you to receive help. Certainly, it's easier to offer help, but can you receive it from others? Can you allow them to serve you? Can you become someone's responsibility even for an hour? No, because you don't want to be a burden, right?

You'll be a burden unless you do for others, unless you constantly do, do do, and do some more. You'd better keep doing because, if you become a burden, you might be rejected... unless you do, do, do.... You might be left out... unless you do, do, do.... You might be so lonely again... unless you do, do, do.... You might not exist... unless you do, do do.... You might have no voice... unless you do, do, do.... You might be in a deeply depressed state again... unless you... do, do, do, do, do!

It is important you know that your values, being, and presence are already worthwhile, and you can give yourself a break. It has been decades of constantly doing for others. You deserve to rest and allow other kind people to serve you as well.

I DON'T TRUST YOU

TRAUMA BODIES HAVE A MONUMENTAL DISTRUST OF others. Even if we truly want to believe we trust others, we don't. The heart wants to trust, but the trauma brain doesn't. Deep down, on an almost cellular level, the familiar alertness is alive and keeps reminding us of the myriad of possibilities that they will betray us.

Our mistrust of others is always simmering in our minds. Trauma doesn't just erase our trust in others, it causes us to constantly question and doubt the people we are with. The truth is, that person on the other end is also going through a lot to be with us. You might have an excellent partner, companion, or friend, and yet you deprive that person of fully receiving you.

Trauma survivors are the most complex beings, and it's a wonder why the people in our lives aren't bored, fed up, and insulted by the level of mistrust we have for them. We constantly keep them at a safe distance, never fully giving them access to ourselves, our minds, our dreams, and our thoughts.

Creating this distance is how we stay safe. We want them to stay where we've placed them and to never expect to be fully embraced in our lives. We believe they're probably plotting something; we can feel it coming. It's almost offensive how little we trust others.

The reality is, if our partners or friends did the same to us, we would be offended. We know they don't deserve it, and yet our survival brains keep scanning and waiting for the other shoe to drop.

OF COURSE YOU WILL DIE

IN THE TRAUMA MIND, EVERYONE IS ABOUT TO DIE. Maybe it will happen now, or in the next second. It will be a sudden death, during a casual, normal evening. For example, the moment my friends leave my home after a nice dinner filled with laughter and joy, in my mind they die.

Not only will they get hurt—that'd be too easy, too impermanent—they will be brutally killed and disappear because of some unknown evil they will encounter the moment they leave my home. The trauma mind doesn't think, *They're just listening to music in the car, and when they get home, they'll have some more wine, plan their next getaway, and probably have sex.* Although that is what they are most likely to do, the trauma mind only sees them dying in a horrific crash.

You can clearly see them driving on the highway, then being catapulted through the windshield in slow-motion. You can hear the windows shatter and the tires skid, and envision them spread across the highway with their hair full of blood.

Somehow—in your mind—you happen to be at the scene of the car crash, staring at your dead friends. As if envisioning them isn't enough, you're mentally transported right there, beside their car, trying to help, trying to stop traffic, trying to call an ambulance, and trying to hold your dead friend's hand.

Next, you're planning the most beautiful funeral service and giving their eulogy. All of this is happening in the trauma mind while your friends walk down the driveway and you're cleaning up from the evening you just had. There is never a joyful landscape painted in your mind. Instead it's a gruesome portrait of the next potential death.

EMPTY SPACE

AS AN ADULT, THERE IS PLENTY OF UNEXPLAINED emptiness inside of me that, no matter how much I work, shop, eat, drink, network, produce, please, or contemplate, can't be filled. The deficiency of nurturing, love, and protection I experienced during my childhood will always haunt me.

Nothing that adult me does can fill the vastness of neglect and fear my inner child still feels, the emptiness of me. Something is always missing. If I get a break today, I'm sure it will slap me in the face tenfold tomorrow.

I AM SO PERFECT

I MADE MYSELF PERFECT AND INTELLIGENT BECAUSE of my fear of being constantly humiliated and ridiculed by my family members. I wasn't born brilliant, and I was afraid of being mocked by those who told me they were better than me.

As I write this, those same grandiose, entitled narcissists would probably want me to thank them for the perfection and knowledge I gained out of my fear of them.

Damn them.

TRAUMA COUNTRY CLUB

WITH TRANSGENERATIONAL TRAUMA, YOUR FAMILY legacy includes membership into a prestigious trauma club. Let's call it the Trauma Country Club. The legacy of trauma is passed down from both parents' lineages, going back generations, like a burdened badge of honor.

You never asked for it, and yet you gained the privilege of a lifetime membership to a club of members who've all been othered. They — like you — are highly knowledgeable, highly observant, and highly alert. Their level of wit and humor is par excellence.

The same is true for their despair. Like you, they've inherited and acquired survival skills unseen anywhere, except in the Trauma Country Club. It's a lifelong perk, and enrollment is free for legacy members. There's even a committee that determines your membership level based on how compliant, obedient, quiet, people-pleasing and put-together you are.

A Silver-level membership is given to those who exhibit neediness, clinginess, a fear of abandonment, manipulative skill, hypochondria, phobophobia, and pessimism. The club would particularly aim for drama queens and kings, and those with demonstrable skills selling hoarded food and medical supplies on the black market (since we never know when the world might end, we're prepared for it).

The Trauma Country Club also welcomes those with ADHD, OCD, dissociation and numbness, as well as any ruminators to this membership level. Substance abusers, dreamers, wounded poets, visionaries, and artists will also feel safe here.

Gold-level members need to exhibit rigidness, dismissiveness, harshness, coldness, self-reliance, cynicism, workaholism, goal-obsession, perfectionism, and—of course—take an interest in sending subliminal messages through social media that only those tuned-in to the right frequency will understand.

Gold members pay a higher rate since they're already working as venture capitalists, VPs, CEOs, and CFOs. However, Gold membership perks include leading, directing, and commanding lower-level members. You can continue to practice the same oppression inside the club that you witnessed and experienced outside of it. We make sure you stay true to your needs.

The Trauma Country Club Board believes membership provides generous benefits for your overall wellbeing and will put you on the path of never-ending enlightenment and catharsis, eventually.

On certain days, trauma mystics will run our retreats. Our licensed trauma mystics have the highest level of experienced trauma. They're considered special and exhibit all the traits of Gold members plus some unique traits all their own. They run all the plant medicine retreats and know the ancient properties of other sacred plants, which are offered only to members with a special pricing plan.

Eventually, the Trauma Country Club will go public, thanks to our numerous angel investors. You will love it here, so much in fact, you'll never want to leave this club. And, with our lifetime memberships, you don't have to! We realize your ancestors won't like that. But what better way to demonstrate your loyalty to them by carrying on the family legacy of trauma?

What's that? No, no, we're not loyal to trauma; we don't dwell. We just gather together to contemplate our inherited trauma history and teach our descendants to do the same. If you prove yourself worthy of membership, you might find this quite lucrative.

MASTER OF THE UNWANTED

I'M A MASTER OF THE UNWANTED. I'VE HONED SO many tools and weapons to survive, ones I never wanted to have in my life. I bet all my ancestors, those who survived two or three wars in their lifetimes, would be proud of the ways I survived mine—both the literal and internal ones.

I've mastered, improved, and expanded all of my tools to keep up with their legacy of resilience and survival. It seems like this mastery is never complete, but I hope it will end with me and bypass my descendants. I wonder why I didn't get handed the ancestral baton to master a joie de vivre as so many others around me received in their legacy? Can I trade with someone?

Would my ancestors be pissed at how I'm giving up all the years of hypervigilance, resourcefulness, and adaptability? They once said, "For God's sake, you can't betray our family legacy! All for the pretense and fluff of comfortable living? We survived *wars*!"

Hmmm. Yes, I would betray it all in a heartbeat for comfort and peace. If I were to place a want ad, it would read:

Expert in surviving, looking to become an expert in tranquility and cultivating pleasure. The general in me is looking to become sensual, relaxed, and filled with human desire, for just a day. I'm not sure how I'll pay you, but if the planet collapses, search for me. I've been drilled to be ready to aim and fire for decades, so I'm sure you will be in good hands.

The general in me is always alert and ready, full of wisdom and terrible knowledge stored deep in my bones. These bones are so tired. They marched through wars and displacements, completely dismissing the basic need for safety and comfort, making horror seem normal.

These bones survived with a clarity and adaptability that surprised the general himself sometimes. I feel this general in me deserves to take a much-needed day of rest and pleasure. At least for one day.

YOU CAN'T JUST BE THERE

YOU CAN ONLY BE WITH SOMEONE—A FRIEND, A CO-worker, or a partner—when you're doing something for them. You can't allow yourself to just be there. You're convinced that you're only allowed to be with others if you're useful to them.

You secured yourself in this role. Otherwise, your presence wasn't welcomed. To be with someone and take pleasure in enjoying their company, while just sitting there listening and absorbing a positive moment of human existence, is a privilege you've never experienced.

It didn't happen for you growing up. You couldn't sink into those normal experiences because your parents probably didn't either. There was no place where you didn't need to be productive, useful, or doing the right thing. There was no place where you could just enjoy someone's presence and a genuine sense of gratitude and love for one another.

TRAUMA EXPERTISE

MEMBERS OF THE TRAUMA AND PTSD COMMUNITY ARE experts in knowing how to go along with things we don't like. Is anyone hiring for the exquisite skill of immense tolerance for other people's bullshit?

SMILE, AND DON'T
BE A BITCH!

LADIES, HOW MANY TIMES HAVE YOU HEARD THIS? "Why don't you smile? Smile. Smile. Smile! Make sure to smile."

Seriously? What would happen to them if you didn't smile? Would it cause them discomfort? Would they calm their unease by demanding that you smile more?

Did they tell you to be a good girl, to be compliant and pleasing? Was it because if you didn't smile, their authority and manhood might be jeopardized? Their intelligence might be questioned? Perhaps your existence vibrated on the wrong comfort frequency for them?

Do you think if all women were made to smile, they would appear subservient, so men could look bigger and more powerful? If you don't keep smiling, they will call you a bitch. Your mother told you to keep smiling and to pretend that everything was fine, or your father would be upset.

"He works so hard; just keep smiling," she said.

Oh, someone just insulted you at the office by making

a bigoted comment? Keep smiling, so you don't make the boys' club feel emasculated. Sure, they can stare at your breasts and be sleazy toward you. Just smile and keep enabling their abuse of power. Smile, and don't be a bitch!

JUST IN CASE, LET ME MAKE MYSELF READY

IN EVERY ESTABLISHMENT AND VENUE, THE FIRST row of seats and the tables closest to the exit are filled with trauma survivors. The escape route needs to be accessible at all times.

Just in case you are suddenly stricken with illness, have a heart attack, develop explosive diarrhea, or suffocate. Just in case terrorists show up, or a plane crashes into the roof, or—just when you are about to take your first bite—all the gas pipes burst into flames, an escape route needs to be accessible at all times.

WHO GETS TO DECIDE WHO IS A BURDEN?

NO SHOULDERS ARE HEAVIER THAN A CHILD'S WHO was forced to carry the weight of being a burden. You were made to feel like a burden to your parents, to your community, and later to your partner or your country.

But the truth is, it is only their entitled belief that you are a burden. A burden to what, their free time? Their standards? Their decisions? Their noble life?

The reality is those self-absorbed, privileged people are actually a burden for the rest of the world, and ninety percent of us are burdened by them. Welcome to the majority. Who is the real burden, then? Us or them? We know the answer.

They are a burden to us, and to this society, by having the narcissistic audacity to say who gets to be a burden. Curiously, they never think they are. What is in their minds, I wonder? How does that thought process work inside of them, deciding and proclaiming that others are a burden?

Perhaps they think, "You are way too hungry. You go in the burden pile!"

If someone asks how to do something, whether it's filing documents or creating a presentation, they immediately go into the burden pile.

Maybe they say, "Oh, no, we need to include more people of color in our workspace to create diversity. This goes into the burden pile."

Who are these people who get to act as if everyone who isn't like them or is inconveniencing them is a burden? Narcissists, of course, and the privileged one-percenters. That entitlement begins in the nuclear family unit and branches outward to people in cubicles, law enforcement, and the government. It spreads everywhere.

Instead, let's put them in our global inconvenience pile, one that we don't need to address or tend to, one that won't occupy our minds. We're the majority, anyhow.

I'M A YES MAN!

YOU MIGHT THINK I'M COMPLIANT AND EASY TO manipulate, but know this, as a trauma survivor, I can see right through you. Don't think you're entitled to my *yes* and don't underestimate it, either.

I don't give my yes because you earned it. It's a remnant of a still-ingrained survival response, meant to placate my oppressor because saying no was a privilege I didn't have. Saying yes meant I would remain safe, unharmed, and alive.

Saying yes didn't provoke more retaliation and rage toward me. It didn't lead to blood on my face. That experience stays with someone for a long time. So, don't think the person who says yes is blind to their response, and that you can use and abuse it for your benefit.

Don't underestimate my yes. The child in me is still scared, but the adult in me can see through your bullshit like no one else can.

WHAT IS ENLIGHTENMENT?

ONCE YOU REALIZE THAT YOUR FATHER WAS ALWAYS numb, your mother was always enabling, your sibling was dissociative, and you were in people-pleasing mode, you feel good for the first time in a long time. You realize your family was a mess and—poof—the fantasy you built around them evaporates into thin air.

This is a divine moment, when you realize how much of a mess everyone is, especially the ones who were explaining things to you, the smart ones who were preaching about how you should behave, or who you should be by now, the ones who apparently knew best!

In that moment, channeled from a spirit, or from God, you finally see that you're not as bad as they made you think you are. You realize you're actually more normal and more developmentally advanced than they are. You almost feel hopeful, and you stand taller and inhale deeper with this realization.

This fantasy, this illusion you built around your family, how everyone is better than you, disappears in front of your eyes. As you finally see how they are all screwed up with their own trauma responses, the burden lifts and you feel lighter for the first time.

This is a moment of enlightenment. This kind of enlightenment needs to have a definition. It is the moment you realize you are the most normal person in your family, and how truly messed up the rest of them are.

Decades-long illusions of holding your family members in high regard dissipate. Celebrate that moment! Breathe it in deeply. It has been a long time coming.

YES, I PLAN

THE PTSD BRAIN IS ALL ABOUT KNOWING WHAT'S next. It's about being certain of the next thing and—of course—you make this happen by constantly planning. It's your source of safety and your survival strategy.

If anyone is annoying enough to ask you why you can't just be spontaneous, or why you need to plan every detail, just ask them the following:

Did you have to grow up with the uncertainty of whether or not your father would come home and burst into a rage, shouting in your face and hitting more than the furniture? No? Well, I did. That's why my nervous system needs to have certainty and to know what will happen next. So, this is what I've planned for this weekend.

Shut them up and keep yourself safe.

DO NOT FEED OFF ME

PEOPLE WHO DELIBERATELY DECIDE NOT TO TAKE ANY responsibility or accountability for their horrific, ignorant, and harmful behavior are human leeches. Why would they be accountable or responsible when they have you, someone who always takes a disproportionate amount of responsibility for other people's behavior?

You are a black hole into which they can dump an infinite amount of blame and guilt, because someone—usually you—made them upset again, and forced them to act out. It's probably your fault anyway. Like leeches, they will suck your energy and make you feel guilty until you take responsibility for what they did.

"I spent our savings. You're responsible for my losses. It was your idea. Besides, the market is in a recession again."

"I cheated on you. You're responsible because you're the one who forced me to find happiness outside of this relationship."

"I slapped our kid across the face. You made them so loud and spoiled. I work all day to feed you, and I need peace and quiet."

"I raped you. You were sending me mixed signals with all those tight clothes, and you didn't say no. You probably liked it."

"I didn't rent my home to an immigrant family. I'm protecting my community from their pollution and crimes."

"I stole your idea and presented it as mine. I communicate better than you and besides, it's not about the idea, it's about turning it into action. Sorry, not sorry! Your bad!"

They are human leeches. What you don't get is that your hyper-responsibility enables their irresponsibility. They have you, so they can continue to be ignorant and nonchalant. They can get away with it for decades.

What you can do to move out of this cycle is to surround yourself with people who can stand up with you and call out unacceptable behavior. Of course, if the person you're dealing with is dangerous or threatens your life, you need legal support and a system of protection.

Otherwise, surround yourself with honest, direct, and bold people. Share your truth. Share the facts and call a meeting or an intervention. Call all the hyper-responsible friends and normal people you know and set up a casual chat. People who aren't accountable are terrified of being publicly shamed and called-out. So, do just that.

Make sure everyone there stares. Look them in their eyes and let them roast. You can pick human leeches off your skin by publicly shaming them. It's not your responsibility to be accountable for their immoral, unethical, and inhumane behavior.

Look around; protecting human leeches is almost incentivized. Society does this by remaining silent and letting their blood sucking continue, or by insinuating that you failed or provoked the abuser to act out. You didn't.

WE ARE INTROVERTS
FOR A REASON

MY LIFE IS SPENT SCANNING EVERY SPACE AROUND me so I can protect myself. That's why my preferred space is my home, and I bet most trauma survivors feel the same.

Too much survival energy goes into scanning every new situation, assessing all the unfamiliar new faces, cities, streets, crowds, and social events for even the tiniest cue of an oncoming threat.

It's enormously exhausting for the nervous system to be laser-focused and constantly detecting the threat of danger, while simultaneously accumulating enough energy to defend oneself—at any moment—in case of a potential attack. This is what life is like with PTSD. The survival brain is hyperactive and completely drained by this task.

It can't just be switched off and allowed to chill. This is why people with trauma and PTSD are often introverts. So, don't ask any of us to explain why we feel like staying at home. Every abuse survivor is, by default, a homebody. Just give us a break from explaining and respect why we prefer a familiar space.

It's not that we're lazy. We're doing the most exhausting work, twenty-four seven, and thankfully, you don't have to. You can chill or go and enjoy new experiences. You can let me know how it was, but I'll be in the safety of my home.

AM I LOSING IT, OR RELEASING IT?

WHAT IS SO BAD ABOUT LOSING IT? WHO INITIALLY said, "You're losing it. You need to pull yourself together," and who decided that should be the social norm?

Was there a person who said, "Don't show any signs of overwhelm, anxiety, fear, or panic in front of anyone, ever. We are about to play bridge and drink tea. Don't you dare be an inconvenience to us"?

And who is the douchebag who supported that? Who set the bar for how we should express ourselves? Even when someone dear to you dies, you are still expected to pull yourself together, to not lose it. You're shamed by the fact that people are listening and watching.

Screaming and crying will disturb everyone. While your entire body is experiencing shock, overwhelm, trauma, and deep loss, you have to be worried about not disturbing others. You're supposed to protect everyone else while you're falling apart. You conditionally suck it up, shove it down, and don't show it.

It's ingrained in you.

"Look at her, she can't contain herself. She's weak. She's hysterical. Look at him. What a wimp!"

Just read these words again. These words, this attitude, is why panic attacks are scary for people.

"Don't lose it!" is a social demand you had to submit to.

The reason why you are conditioned this way is because the person who witnesses your panic experiences discomfort. It's their lack of education, their selfishness, or their fear.

It's a reminder of their humanity and helplessness, and they don't know what to do with it or with you.

What people need to understand is that when someone is "losing it," it's actually a release, a discharge from their nervous system. (I am not referring to complex mental conditions such as psychotic disorders.)

It's the release of initial shock or overwhelm. Screaming, crying, and shaking are ways the body releases trauma. Allow it to move through you. Do not shut it down, suppress it, or shame it. Otherwise, it will be expressed as a panic attack.

When I'm "losing it," I don't need a strategy, a quick fix, or a plan of action. I don't need to be quiet and wipe my face with a tissue, either. I need to be held so I can cry, wail, scream out loud, moan, or shake.

I need to labor out my overwhelm and you, as my doula, just need to hold my hand, whisper to me gently, and nurture me with your presence. You don't need to fix me. My nervous system is intelligent and will settle down as the release moves through me. It's a natural process in humans and animals. It comes to completion in a safe environment, with safe, supportive people.

When you feel fear and panic, do you want to hide under a blanket or hide in the bathroom while you're hyperventilating, just so you don't disturb your friends? Look at the amount of shame you feel in this state. You feel the need to hide your panic attacks so you don't distress others. In your deepest state of stress, you need to be considerate about not distressing your friends, relatives, or neighbors, and need to stay calm and collected so you don't get labeled as the "crazy one."

This is exactly what makes people crazy. You hold it in,

hold it in, hold it in, and then you have a nervous break-down. Seriously. I don't want to "power through" and stay put. I need to release, to be human in my fear and to be fragile when it's happening. I need to be accepted in an environment where I will be held when I am overwhelmed and having a panic attack.

We need to make a club of people you can call, just so you can lose it. The Lose It club will welcome you, hold you, and understand you, so that, instead of holding everything tight, you can loosen up and let it out!

Other folks will run from you. Who wants to be with the crazy one, the one who loses it, the unpredictable one? Use that in your favor; they can't help you much, anyhow.

So, next time someone violates your boundaries, just say, "I'm about to lose it. My craziness is coming up! It's coming!" and watch with delight as they quickly silence themselves and retract, as if anything they say or do will detonate you.

They certainly won't inconvenience themselves by watching you lose it, so they might even start washing the dishes or take the kids on a walk, so they aren't in your pres-ence. Enjoy the free time and do not be scared or ashamed, not ever again, about "losing it."

YOU DON'T NEED
TO FORGIVE

THERE'S THIS BELIEF THAT YOUR NERVOUS SYSTEM
will relax, that you will heal, and that you'll be a good person
if you forgive the people who hurt you. It's a spiritual thing
to forgive. God is forgiving, so it's expected of you to forgive,
too. You're the bigger person if you forgive.

When I hear this, I feel like someone just insulted me. I'm
told to forgive my perpetrator, so I can feel better and my nervous system can regulate. So many things are wrong with this.

Some people do not deserve grace and forgiveness. They
deserve justice.

If I forgive my perpetrators, I abandon and betray the
horror that was done to me for more than a decade. I would
abandon that fourteen – or twenty-one year-old, still living
alert and vigilant inside of me. I would betray myself, and
that is something I will never do. It was enough that the
system and the people who were supposed to protect me
betrayed me, I won't do it to myself as well.

This imposed belief in forgiveness for your abuser is non-
sense. It's yet another piece of mindful bullshit that people
with trauma and PTSD can't digest. It's the same as the
unhelpful advice to not be angry.

"You need to forgive them!" they say. Are they shaming
me because they're afraid I won't be a noble and graceful
person to someone who deeply violated my human rights?
Why do they care? I will never forgive, and I don't have to in
order to heal.

Were they in my shoes? Were they begging for their life
when they had a gun pressed to their forehead? Were they

held to the ground while their underwear was ripped off? I don't think so. Forgive? It's an insult to hear this, especially from prominent "gurus" and mental health professionals.

I will never betray myself by forgiving my abusers. I believe in accepting what happened. I believe in grieving, in mourning lost innocence. I believe in the protection of human rights and dignity, and in seeking justice, not forgiveness for human scum.

I don't believe in holding grudges, but rather in the process of accepting and grieving what was done to us. I no longer feel anger over what was done to me, but there is anger when I hear, "It's better to forgive."

I think those who are preaching forgiveness are dissociated or have not been deeply wounded, as millions of others were. As for myself and those millions, we do not want to forgive—not ever.

LET ME PREPARE YOU SO YOU CAN PROCESS

HOW MANY OF YOU ARE COMING FROM FAMILIES THAT prepared you for making your own decisions or, at minimum, considered you in any of the decisions they made that impacted your life? How many of you were allowed time to process your feelings and experiences?

Did your parents invite your opinion about the decisions that affected you? Did they consider your input and give you time to form your thoughts? No, because this doesn't happen in families experiencing trauma.

You were raised to not process, or even think you were entitled to take time to process. Time for processing and being taught how to evaluate things from your own experience doesn't exist in trauma. Time for processing is a privilege.

Did anyone ever tell you they will give you time to think? Did they say you could analyze the situation, talk with your therapist, reflect, and process? Did they assure you that they would patiently wait for your response, and although they might not agree with it, they would still respect your decision?

Seriously. Did that ever happen to you growing up, or even now? That's a privilege I know many of us wish we had.

Imagine a parent saying, "Son, we need to talk to you. We are planning to uproot your life and immigrate to a new country next year. Would you prefer to stay home and continue your life here, or come with us? We will process this big decision with our counselor and priest, and we want to make sure your thoughts are considered. You are precious to us. We have a year to prepare and transition into a new life."

I have never heard of this happening in a family with trauma. What I did hear and experience was my father slamming the front door and shouting, "You have five minutes to pack your things. Only bring underwear, two shirts and pants, and nothing else! Did you hear me? They might come for us! Don't you dare call your friends or say anything to anyone. Pack now, and fast! *Move!*"

Choice? Processing? Consideration? Preparation?

Did you hear, "Son, have you considered taking another route in establishing your career? Have you considered pursuing law instead of art? We already have a stable business. Your intelligence and skills will be incredibly valuable to us," from your parents?

Or did they say, "I won't have a daydreamer in my house, and certainly not someone who will ruin the family legacy!

This is what I did, and what your grandfather did. If you want to live your dream, I will make sure the family cuts you off—don't look at your mother! You will not embarrass us and live out of my pocket," in order to control you?

Were you told, "My daughter, I'm sad you're going to spend the holidays with your partner. It would be wonderful if you could join us, but if you choose to be with your partner, know that I respect your choice. Let me know when you decide," by your parents?

Most likely, what you actually experienced was hearing, "You know we don't have long to live, and your mom has had this holiday planned for a long time. The memories you lose with us will always be on your conscience. It's up to you."

Did anyone say, "I'm frustrated with what happened. I see we have conflicting views on the choice we need to make. Can we set up a day and time to talk, and if we need outside help, let's find it. I don't want this to be an obstacle for us," in the midst of a difficult decision?

Or was it, "Don't tell me to calm down! You're making me crazy. It's your fault I get so mad. You made me do it. Stop overreacting! I didn't even touch your face. Keep pushing your agenda and I will leave you. The kids are staying with me, and don't you dare call your friends," in the heat of an argument?

Were you prepared for, considered, valued, respected, and given time to process? There is no such thing when you live a life filled with neglect, abuse, and trauma.

Choice, consideration, the time to process and decide, and having respect for your opinion and wishes, have never been options in families with trauma. Never. You need to listen, obey, follow, and immediately agree, with no option to think or say, "Let me get back to you once I consider my options," or "Let me process what you just told me." That privilege never comes in a life with trauma.

CRAZY ONE

ARE YOU CONCERNED ABOUT HOW YOUR FEELINGS will be perceived by others, or that you might be called crazy? Are you suppressing your experiences, feelings, reality, and everything else meaningful to you, just so you won't be labeled a drama queen or someone who doesn't have their life together?

What you feel inside of your body is provoked from the outside, but trauma happened to you and inside of you. It's your experience. It's what happened to you, to your identity, and to your biology. What you feel inside of your body and mind is yours. It's valid. It's a part of your story, and of your life.

Who gets to judge and decide how much you should or should not feel, what you're allowed to express, and in what increments?

No one from the outside can know what your internal experience is. They can't know your pain, or your symptoms. How could they? Do they live inside of your body? It's only you who knows what it's like in your body. Your experience is yours.

I wish there was some kind of device where you could place all of those judgmental friends, family members, and know-it-alls inside of your body to experience your emotional state for just one hour. If you could stick them in that place where anguish, terror, pain, and loneliness are all combined, how would they feel then?

When they scream out for help, in fear and pain, with heart palpitations and sweat collecting around their face, just tell them, "Why are you stuck in the past? God, you are *so* sensitive. Can't you just meditate or learn to manifest? You're being dramatic. You have a great life. Why do you always make a big deal about everything? Far worse things have happened to me, and look how I turned out. Don't pout. I just read a book about it. All you have to do is think positively! Now, I'm going to the gym. You stay where you are. Isn't it nice in this place? Take a look around. You only have fifty-nine minutes left!"

I wonder if they will ever think or say you're crazy again!

YOU NEED TO DESERVE IT

DO YOU DESERVE TO TAKE TIME? TO PAUSE? TO BE happy? To laugh? To express your own voice? To eat? To sing? You probably feel you need to earn all of it. You need to be deserving of feeling joy, of feeling alive. If you or your ancestors were enslaved, or sent to forced labor camps, or lived under oppression, you may have heard these words.

Your oppressor would say, "You deserve it when I say you do."

You and your ancestors listened to that voice for a long time, so it sunk into each of your bones. You truly believe you need to deserve to own, to express, and to act on your basic human rights because you don't have any worth or value. You believe you need to wait for someone else's permission.

Do you really need to earn the right to feel joy, or to rest, or to be worthy of having or feeling anything? Do you really need to deserve the right to express your needs?

The notion that anyone has to deserve fundamental things

like safety, nourishment, love, freedom, and the right to make their own choices is abuse. A bird doesn't have to earn its wings to fly, it just does. A flower doesn't have to deserve to grow, it just does. And you don't have to deserve to have your needs met, you are entitled to have them met because you exist and you had innate value the moment you were born.

MAKE A CHOICE FOR ME. GIVE ME PERMISSION. THEN I CAN LIVE.

YOU LEARNED YOU DIDN'T HAVE THE RIGHT TO MAKE a choice. You normalized accepting other people's choices instead of your own. You were never allowed to make a choice. Even years after you left your family home, or escaped oppression and the violation of your human rights, you still feel like you don't have the right to make a choice.

Somehow, you still obediently wait for others to decide for you. You just need to be compliant, right? Even if one day you are brave enough to make a choice or dream about something, you won't start it unless you receive permission from someone else.

The fact is, that permission is never coming because no one spends that much time thinking about other people. People are wrapped up in their own traumas and issues, and toxic people will move on to their next victim. You are a fully functioning adult, and you're still obediently waiting for permission to start living.

And you wonder where your life went? It disappeared waiting for your caregivers, maybe your father or your mother, to give you permission. Or maybe it vanished because of an abusive partner or an oppressive government. You continue to wait, and eventually, you'll die in the same place, waiting.

THE TRAUMA HERO'S JOURNEY. LUKE BECOMES A JEDI

THE HERO'S JOURNEY IS A COMMON STORYLINE where the hero leaves home to defeat dangerous adversaries and comes home transformed. Those who are dealing with their trauma every day are facing a hero's journey, sometimes multiple times in a day. Let me break it down for you into the three stages of the hero's journey, the template on which all superhero movies are based.

STAGE ONE: DEPARTURE

In the Departure stage, also known as "the Call to Adventure," the hero leaves the security of their home and familiar surroundings and goes into the unknown.

As a trauma survivor, how does it feel, every single day, to wake up knowing you have to face the world around you? How does it feel when you need to turn the doorknob and leave your home in order to face people at work or at school? How does it feel when everything in you just wants to curl back in bed and hide?

You can almost feel it in your stomach, that nauseated quality of fear, struggle, and unease. Every day, when you open the door to leave your home, you are entering the anti-gravity of the unknown, and for a trauma body, that takes enormous effort. It's an adventure you don't want to take, and yet you are embarking upon it.

---

* Joseph Campbell, a professor and author credited with popularizing the idea of the hero's journey in his 1949 book, *The Hero with a Thousand Faces*, called this stage the "Call to Adventure."

STAGE TWO: INITIATION

In this phase, the hero faces a succession of hardships and tribulations. The hero's journey is dangerous. Battle, skill, and strife put the hero to the test. The hero may not succeed in every deed, but they must persevere. Throughout the initiation stage, the hero will encounter friends, villains, and even mentors who offer magical assistance.

In this stage, you walk out your door and know you'll be tested in numerous battles. You need to face traffic, loud sounds, your commute. You already have your go-to tools to help you breathe through possible panic attacks in your car, or you have an excuse prepared in case you need to leave the meeting and run to the bathroom to hide your anxiety.

Throughout all of these constant battles in your head, there is also a chronic fear that you will be discovered as inadequate due to your mental state. You frantically worry about how badly you will embarrass yourself. You think about how you will be judged and shamed in front of your colleagues and friends. Everyone around you looks like an enemy, not an ally or a mentor. Not in a trauma body.

With a seemingly supernatural power that resides in you — not outside of you as in the traditional hero's journey — you pull an enormous amount of strength, resiliency, and skill from the depths of your bones, all of which you keep denying you have.

You pull that strength out like a blazing sword and march through every trial and tribulation of the day, carrying it high. In a trauma body, you experience dozens of these heroic moments, every single day. Dozens of times a day, you overcome your trauma tribulations. And even with all of that battle armor weighing you down, you still manage to deliver great work, because what trauma survivor isn't a perfectionist and excellent employee?

You will even chat with others. You will politely nod and listen to someone's self-absorbed story about their trip to Mexico, and you will be of service to anyone who needs you throughout the day.

STAGE THREE: RETURN

After enduring the difficulties and tribulations of the quest, the hero returns home in the third stage. However, the hero has changed. Through the maturing process of the dangerous encounter, an inward shift has occurred. Luke has become a Jedi and has made peace with his past. Neo accepts his fate and frees himself from the constraints of the Matrix. When the hero comes home, they are recognized, appreciated, even exalted, for the feats they've accomplished and the battles they've fought.

Pause and read the preceding paragraph one more time. You are the hero, the jedi, the one who escaped the matrix. You have returned home after the tremendous hardship of a scary adventure, and you survived. You made it. What you keep denying is the resiliency and strength you display to do even seemingly simple things, like get through the day.

What's missing is the validation that you, like any returning hero, deserve after surviving every single day. If that is not heroic, what is it? Is it just fluff and pretense? Is it posing and faking smiles on Instagram? What is heroic? Who is a hero?

You are living with trauma and keeping yourself going, every single day. That is the mark of a hero. I see deep strength, will, resiliency, and monumental capabilities in you. Acknowledge what you have. Give yourself the validation, the recognition, you deserve.

Remember how Luke became a Jedi and found peace with his past? Imagine that Luke returned home with a magical elixir. Imagine you have this elixir, and it is your acknowledgment that you are not your past. You are not what has been done to you. You get to recognize the hero you are now.

In my eyes, every single trauma survivor is a Jedi who goes on a hero's journey every day. How can you not admire that? I salute you. Can you take credit for yourself? Can you validate what you go through, every day?

There are millions, if not billions of people who are on the hero's journey with you. Others with PTSD and trauma are walking that journey, too. You are not alone.

At the end of each day, look for micro-shifts of change and transformation inside of you. A moment of realization will come, and you will allow yourself to have pride because you are an amazing hero.

IDEA TO MAKE YOUR MILLIONS, BABE

HOW DO YOU KNOW WHAT HEALTHY BEHAVIOR IS when you come from a lineage of female servants and enraged fathers? Is there any school, membership, retreat, self-guided course, or mastermind group for it? Can you provide me with the exact tools for healthy adult living? Can you direct me to a place where I can learn how to keep my agency, because those tools were never given to me?

It's not just me asking these questions. It's a big niche group—maybe ninety percent of our population. Please, all you digital nomads, entrepreneurs, million-dollar mastermind babes, set up a school for us.

Set up a school where I can lose the tendency to obediently say yes to others and serve them at the snap of their fingers because of my deep fear that a man will scream at me if I don't. But, be forewarned, I can't be accountable if, at some point in the workshop or retreat, a century of pent-up rage bursts out of my bones and I become my father.

FIGHT THAT URGE

You want to run away when you can't breathe
in a restaurant? Fight that urge!

You want to say, "F—you, what you did is abuse" to
the person who hurt you? Fight that urge!

You want to feel pleasure? Fight that urge!

You want to sing? Fight that urge!

You want to be silly? Fight that urge!

You want to express yourself, write a book,
put a song out? Fight that urge!

Brace it, compress it, depress it, and do
not express it! Fight that urge!

Because, what will people think of you?

JUDGE ME NOT

YOU ASKED ME—WITH A TONE OF JUDGMENT AND frustration—why my fridge was overflowing with food. I explained it was because I spent many years of my life hungry, waiting in line to eat. The night I told you this, I lost you forever. My life was too uncomfortable for you.

You lost your ground to play the trendy environmental minimalist. You lost your right to judge me and act more spiritually advanced. You pretended, your entire adult life, to be some kind of an ascetic, casually ignoring the inherited money you can always swim back to.

So, go find someone like you. Someone who you can join together with in a false pretense of advanced spirituality, with a fat bank account that you can try to hide with your ripped clothes and self-deprived lifestyle.

My fridge will always spill over with decadent pleasures. It is a reminder to my hungry teen-self of all the love she can receive from the adult me. It is a reminder that she will never be deprived enough to stand hungrily in a food line again.

EXCLUDED FOR FAMILY CONVENIENCE

DO YOU WONDER WHAT'S WRONG WITH YOUR FAMILY? How many times have you done everything to adjust your life and your plans just to fit around theirs, and how many times have they done the same for you? How many times have you been excluded from their plans when it comes to celebrations, reunions, dinners, or BBQs?

How many times did you say that you understood and it was okay? How many times did they understand you? Maybe they accidentally confessed over a phone call that they were having a big gathering and excluded you, again, for family convenience. How many times were you left out of planning parties or celebrations — overlooked, as if you were less important? Or even expected not to come?

Overlooked, as if you were less important.

"She won't get upset. She will understand. She is so far away anyway; why bother? She is too busy anyhow."

Isn't that a convenient way to be excluded, and such an easy justification? Where does that leave you? In pain, heartbroken, and angry.

They certainly made an effort for their friends. How could your own family overlook you? You carry their name, you might have a room in their home, you have a history together, and you were likely seated at their dinner table every night for years. You were not invisible.

The irony is that they get offended if you even try to do something fun on your own. How dare you try, and how dare you not adjust your plans so they can come along with you.

Funerals are a different story, though. When someone in

the family dies, even a distant relative, I bet they will wait for you and obligingly adjust to your schedule, so you can bear all the responsibility and be of service to them.

They will even postpone burying their loved one for as long as possible so you can come and arrange everything, like calling funeral homes, picking out the urn or coffin, writing the eulogy, ordering flowers, contacting relatives and friends, and securing a location for the services. You're good at that, so of course, they will include you. When you make their lives easier, you will be considered, invited, and included in the family.

"Here comes the somber, agile planner who can take care of all the funeral stuff. She needs to be there. Trauma, death, terminal cancer, mourning—she is good with that. Parties and celebrations, not so much. She is the serious sibling, the sibling of death."

Afterward, they will probably plan a weekend getaway at a retreat to rest and recuperate from the funeral, and with a concerned look in their eyes, they will send you home because you are needed somewhere else. Another crisis is waiting for you.

They will pick up their suitcases for a spa weekend, and you will be conveniently overlooked again because you simply do not belong with the family you were born into, unless a crisis happens.

MY NEEDS CANNOT EASILY BE SPOKEN

I LEARNED TO EXPLAIN MY WANTS AND NEEDS AS IF I'm going into battle. Armed, alert, ready to push back or submit, and even pretend I'm sick if necessary. Migraines are always handy.

I've preplanned what I will say. I've rehearsed my power words, prepared my argument, and I will fight, manipulate, or defend myself if I have to — even if all I want to do is spend a couple hours on my own over the weekend and skip family brunch.

It's as if there is no other way around it than to justify and fight for a simple need. Fight for it. Fight. Fight. Fight. Do you feel this way, as if you really need to earn it, sweat for it, experience a racing heart, a panic attack, anger, and a stiff neck? Or do you need to become an octopus, with a genius, insidious plan you slowly wrap around someone like tentacles so they'll submit to your basic need to spend a little time alone.

That comes from trauma. You were conditioned to fight for every single need growing up because you were dismissed, stonewalled, ridiculed, shamed or even punished if you needed something. Now as an adult, you keep defending your needs as if you don't have any right to have them. You act as if you always need permission from others. That is the result of trauma.

TRAUMA LIFE

WHAT SEEMS SO CASUAL AND EFFORTLESS FOR others, is a source of enormous anxiety and pressure for me. Leaving home, commuting, going to dinners, taking vacations, attending parties, hosting get-togethers, buying gifts, presenting something to a group—all of it takes enormous preparation, thinking, sleepless nights, sweaty hands, IBS, nausea, and panic attacks.

And yet, I do it. I keep torturing myself on my own now. It seems it is more important for me to keep the sadistic self-punishing legacy going in my family than it is to preserve my wellbeing.

DO NOT TAKE
ANY SPACE!

WHEN YOU LEARNED YOUR PRESENCE MADE THE people you lived with upset, angry, or silent, a deep and toxic trauma shame was born. You spent your life feeling as if your presence would ruin other people's moods, just by showing up.

Your identity becomes bothersome and wrong, you are someone who upsets others. You learn the safest way to exist is to not take up any space. Even riding in an elevator by yourself feels like taking up too much space, so you move to the corner in case others step inside. Your whole life is spent in that corner of the elevator, where your parents put you in the first place. You never dare to move closer to the control panel, to breathe in deep enough for your lungs and chest to expand; you never take up any more space than necessary. That is how damaging trauma shame is.

ONLY MARRYING TRAUMA SURVIVORS

SELFISH, SELF-ABSORBED PEOPLE NEED TO SUR-round themselves with trauma survivors. Maybe on a dating app they should write that they're only look ng to date and hopefully marry trauma survivors. The worse the trauma, the better.

It would be a match made in heaven. The self-absorbed partner's needs would be taken care of before they even became aware of them. The trauma survivor would always be five steps ahead of them. The selfish partner wouldn't need to do anything to help, serve, or support their partner with trauma.

Why? Because trauma survivors are the most self-reliant people in the world. They won't ask for help, not even when they're on their deathbed. Even then, they will make sure to dress themselves in presentable clothing so no one needs to change them for the funeral service, which they already paid for twenty years ago.

They will make sure they leave fresh fruit trays and juice in the fridge so no one gets hungry when they're called to take them to the funeral home. Even then, with their last breath, their trauma mind will hope no one needs to do anything for them, because they don't want to be an inconvenience to anyone. The trauma mind thinks:

They must be bored with me by now. I'm going to die lying here doing nothing for them. I should keep talking until my last breath so they're entertained and I'm not a burden to them. Maybe I can play my Spotify playlist that I prepared specifically for when I die, so when they're about to call the funeral home to take my body, the vibe will be relaxing for everyone. I'll do anything to help, just as long as I'm not a burden, even when I'm cold and dead.

6

OPPRESSION
AND ABUSE
OF POWER

BEFORE THEY
GOT RID OF ME

ALL OF MY GIVING, ALL OF MY SERVING, ALL OF MY people-pleasing came from a need to be accepted just a bit longer. I knew in the core of my being that any day, any hour, any second, I would become unwanted, rep aced, and uninvited. My desperation grew louder as others' acceptance of me waned, and I could feel that the moment of my abandonment was approaching.

All the excellent work, the overtime, the over-delivery, the over-appeasement, the frantic effort for cecades—all of it—came from living in anticipation of being rejected and desperately needing to be accepted just a bit longer, just one more day, before I would be abandoned again.

I had to make myself valuable so people would need me longer. The more they needed me, the less chance I would be cast aside that day. I lived in this space of fear, always reaching for a bit more acceptance before the inevitable time when they would get rid of me.

I WILL NOT EDUCATE YOU

I HAVE ZERO TOLERANCE FOR IGNORANCE FROM those who live in a place of privilege. On many occasions, people who pretended to care casually asked me to educate them about oppression. Probably because I am white, it made them more comfortable to ask me, rather than a person of color who survived similar experiences of war and genocide.

They wanted me to spend my time educating them about oppression over dinner. Really? They have all the resources imaginable, but they have made zero effort to learn and educate themselves on their own, and yet they feel comfortable enough to ask me—in my free time—to use my energy and knowledge, and to recall my trauma memories to educate them. They do this as if it checks the box for their required human and civic duties.

As if asking gives them an excuse, a way to say they tried and made a micro-effort. They can say, "I asked her. She's a therapist. She was in wars, sent off to be a child soldier, lived as a refugee, was an undocumented farm worker, and was homeless, but she didn't want to talk about it with me. So, I will have to keep being ignorant. It's not my fault that she didn't help me. Time to go back to my winery and see what label I can make for my new fancy bottle of rosé."

I will not stop my life for a moment to educate privileged people so they can pat themselves on the back as if they made an effort.

ABUSE OF POWER

NOTHING MAKES YOU DOUBT YOUR VALUE AND SENSE of worthiness like someone in a position of power implying that you are an outcast, that they see you as filth. Who do you turn to when the authority figures around you tell you that you are less?

Where is your place of value then? Where do you go to nurture your importance and mirror your worthiness? What's even more damaging is that in an abuse of power, there is often no restitution or reconciliation of any kind to help you wash away the humiliation of being devalued and dehumanized.

Further, it is insulting that if reconciliation and restitution is offered, it's typically by those who abused their power in the first place, and who took decades of precious time between their golf swings and cocktail hours to educate themselves and decide when it was time to make a pathetic attempt at amends. The ones who committed crimes against humanity got to decide. Yuck.

FRANTIC PERFECTIONISM

Faster, faster, faster!

Now, now, now!

Prove it, prove it, prove it!

Only the best, only the best, only the best!

See me now? See me now. See me now!

I am working hard! I am working super hard!

I know how! I really know how!

One more time! Not a problem! One
more time! One more time!

Do not pause! Do not pause! No
pauses! Do not take a break!

Hold your breath; you need to prove yourself all over again!

Hold your breath, and keep holding it, every
single minute of every single day!

I know I can do it. I will do it. I have to
do it! I cannot take a break!

They will decide if I am worthy of them.

They will decide if I belong with them!

I *need* them to approve of me

Them, them, them, them, them!

Not me, not me, not me, there is no *me*!

It is my existence in their hands; how can't you see it?

I am holding my breath and doing my best to be accepted,
even if it's only for twenty seconds of their presence!

OPPRESSED

OPPRESSED PEOPLE ARE CONDITIONED TO THINK THE
only way they can belong, be accepted, seen, or appreciated is by doing their best, all the time. It never occurs to the
oppressed person that others will receive them and appreciate them for who they are, or that they will respect their
humanity, the simple kindness and worth of their being.

Growing up, they didn't witness or experience appreciation, nor were they welcomed as a human being. They were
forced to be a human doing. Humanness was punished. Going
above and beyond meant safety, at least in the moment. It
meant that as long as they were needed, they would stay alive.

There are so many people who have experienced this. Immigrants, enslaved people, migrant farm workers, impoverished persons, people of various ethnicities, skin colors, and sexualities that deviate from the standard white cisgender heterosexual "norm." There are so many humans who were and are othered.

This is how perfectionists and people with severe work ethics are born. They are trauma survivors. They never stop doing, as long as they receive a silent nod of approval and reassurance. They do this hoping they won't be ostracized or exiled from the group, like they were by their society or country.

The trauma of oppression makes you a master of many skills. Mastery is not achieved because of some natural-born ambition or talent, but a desperate fear of being shamed and an innate need to belong and survive. Receiving recognition and acceptance proves that they matter and exist as a human.

For that twenty seconds of appreciation from others, we will do eighty-hour work weeks, over and over again. Oppressed trauma body is a place where laser-focused delivery, masterfulness, and frantic fear mixed with deep exhaustion exists twenty-four seven.

So, if you see a perfectionist at work, or someone who is working exceptionally hard, please take a moment to share kind words and look in their eyes. You will see the reflection of deep humanness and lifelong gratitude.

WHO DO YOU
TURN TO?

WHO HOLDS YOU IN YOUR DESPAIR WHEN THE SPACE around you is hostile, when no one is safe, when your body rejects you, and when all traces of hope are gone? Who do you turn to? When God or faith was never modeled as a source of comfort and trust? Who do you turn to?

You turn to your ancestors. Hundreds, maybe even thousands, of years ago, they survived, even though living is so hard. You, the descendant of those survivors, are still here, surviving. So, turn to them. Feel them behind you. Lean into them, breathe into them, sink into them. You survived. You have them as your resource. Breathe, just breathe into them, and then walk with them, step by step.

See the sky, see the trees, see the water, hear the birds, and lean on your ancestors. They sit in your bones. Feel the strength of all you had to endure, and their support in your spine. You will recover. Even in our deepest isolation, we are not alone.

Your ancestors will encourage you to seek help. They will hold you in your despair, and they will remind you of all the resiliency you carry inside of you. Remember that, like them, you survived.

BURDEN OF WISDOM

I would rather have no trace of wisdom than
have wisdom born out of pain and survival.

DO I?

Do I have depth to see? Yes I do.

Do I have incredible resiliency? Yes I do.

Do I have knowledge? Yes I do.

Do I have strength enough to witness a
nation's gore and pain? Yes I do.

Do I know how to survive? Yes I do.

Do I have joyfulness? No I don't, and I never will.

Do I have innocence? No I don't, and I will never get it back.

Do I have ease and rest? No I don't, nor will my children.

THE ENTREPRENEUR
IN YOU

THE EXPERIENCE OF VIOLENCE CREATES AN IMPRINT that causes you to look down and listen to authority figures. In the body, there's a repulsion and revolt against working in any structured system where you have to report to someone. Everything in you wants to run away from it, and yet there is this conditioned obedience toward the system.

If you wonder why you are unhappy working in a bank, in a school, an insurance company, or anywhere structured, it's because your body recalls the authoritarian, violent, and screaming figures you had to report to and hide from in the past.

In a nutshell, that is your raging father or another abusive figure, who, for a child, represents a system—the family system—that you had to listen to and report to. Your raging abuser is always a cloud above your head, even when you are in your forties.

Your boss or your manager feels exactly like the authoritarian figure you experienced before. Even if you have a decent boss, when you make a small mistake and they call you in to discuss it, it can produce anxiety, fear, and sweat in your body.

Your body recalls abusive memories from the past and screams in resistance. It remembers when you were summoned, yelled at, and violated. That is why trauma survivors thrive on being self-employed and running their own businesses.

It gives you a sense of autonomy, agency, and integrity. It gives you a place where you make the decisions, and where you can collaborate with your people, your team, and your adoptive family. It is a place where you always look up and never down, because there is no one above you to be upset with you.

When you work for yourself, you build an environment where your nervous system feels safe. There, you flourish and achieve more than you would if you were still working in someone else's system, being tamed and constricted, and fighting nausea in the morning, every single day.

PERFORMANCE, NOT LOVE

I COME FROM PARENTS AND A LINEAGE WHERE PERformance and strength were more valued than acts of service through love. In my upbringing, vulnerability was condemned and performance was praised. I was taught to hide love out of the fear that my strength would be taken away. Love wasn't seen as a strength.

I was taught that I could only have one way of showing strength, and not another. I was deprived, and therefore, I risked depriving my own children of seeing my love and the delicate beauty of my tenderness. I lived in fear that if I showed my love, I would lose it, that somehow it would be taken away from me and that I would be left embarrassed.

When my grandparents' oppressors saw how much they loved their kids, they took or killed their kids away, so that my grandparents would suffer more. They did this to kill human will, so they would obey and work harder.

My family learned never to show their love, and to force themselves to replace that tender expression with pure strength and performance in order to move forward. Those qualities were born from the fear that the ones they loved would be taken away. Showing love meant losing love. Showing love meant heartbreak.

Like me, your lineage of strength and performance was born out of your ancestor's desire to protect their loved ones. What legacy will you leave for your descendants? Do you still live in fear that your oppressors will punish you if, for just a moment, you clearly show how much you love the people in your life?

WHEN THE SYSTEM SPITS YOU OUT

THE SYSTEM—INCLUDING LAW ENFORCEMENT, PRO-fessional sports, healthcare workers and the military—takes you in. You trust the system. You're devoted to it.

You're invested in it. You work harder than the rest, remain above the norm, and stay loyal to it. It's almost like— if not even better than—family. And then you burn out and develop PTSD because of that same system's ignorance about the wellbeing of its people.

The system is barely trauma-informed, and almost no one is trauma-trained. They send you to exposure therapy, which escalates your PTSD even more. Then doctors look at you with confusion, annoyance, cluelessness, or helplessness.

In that system, everyone in a position to help you has failed you. The president or CEO has failed you, HR, VPs, managers, counselors, and doctors all failed you; and your PTSD makes you feel like you've failed them.

The system spits you back out—maybe with benefits, but maybe not—and you're left in isolation, on your own, trying to figure out what's happening to you and how to move on from one day to the next.

You feel used, betrayed, and rejected. I hope that after you read this, you will find a therapist who's trained in PTSD and trauma recovery.

I hope that some VPs and CEOs will read this and wake up, add full trauma care to the system, center care and compassion for their employees, and stop being ignorant about the mental health of the people who are the backbone of the system they control.

DARE TO MAKE
A MISTAKE

IN YOUR FAMILY, WERE YOU ALLOWED TO MAKE A MIS-
take and casually brush it off, knowing no fuss would be
made, or at least no painful and shameful consequences
would follow?

Or, were you beaten up, slapped, yelled at, and shamed
when you made a mistake growing up? When someone
has always screamed at you when you make a mistake,
how daring and curious can you be later on in life? Did their
threats and punishments set you up to explore, learn new
things, and challenge yourself in life?

No. Of course not.

So, what message was imprinted on you, and on your
ancestors? If you make any mistakes, you will be beaten up
and hurt. You will lose your job. You will not be able to provide for your family.

Can you dare to make a mistake? It's not an option when
you're in the hands of your abuser, a colonizer, or an oppressor. It's too costly to make a mistake. This is why BIPOC and
invisible minorities are not seen as explorers, trendsetters,
or scientists, or at least as people who — like anyone else —
change jobs, move to new locations, or work in career fields
where curiosity, trying, and failing are the norm.

You and your ancestors could never make a mistake.
Making mistakes equals being assaulted and ostracized, and
that is why you stick to what is known, what is steady, and
what you have perfected to the core, so you and your family
will not be harmed.

Even if that means you never change jobs, never learn a

new skill, and never move to a different place, you will not dare expose yourself to the possibility of making any mistake, not ever again.

You have also transferred those high survival expectations to your kids.

Don't you dare make mistakes, kids, you tell them with your eyes, your words, your body language. *I can't bear to watch your dignity get taken away!*

Or your life, your ancestors will whisper in your ear.

WHAT PEEKS HAVE YOU BEEN SNEAKING?

DO YOU WALK DOWN THE STREET, PEEKING CAUtiously at others' faces? Not with a full, open gaze, but just sneaking looks with your neck stiff and braced, as if it's not safe to look at them or hold their gaze. You don't know what might jump out and come at you. Maybe your whole body feels tense as you pass people on the street.

Do you sneak a peek at other people's hands when you are sitting in the movies or in meetings, cautiously aware that they might do something to you? Do other people see hands as a source of discomfort and unexplainable threat?

What about shoes left in the hallway at the entrance of a door? Do you sneak a peek at them, cautiously looking for the pair of shoes that will cause a twisting pain in your stomach the moment you see them?

What prevents you from fully seeing other people's

faces? Is it the constant fear that someone's face will erupt in rage and their hands will swing toward you? Does seeing a certain pair of shoes remind you of someone who harmed you in the past? What peeks have you been sneaking?

THE COLLECTIVE CRAZINESS OF COLLECTIVE TRAUMA

IN COLLECTIVE TRAUMA, THERE'S A VAST LANDSCAPE of numbness and denial. You survived communism, wars, slavery, colonialism, genocide, and the injustice of what happened in front of your eyes to your child, to your brother, to your sister, to your being, to your ethnic group, all by dismissing your own and each other's reality.

You dismissed it, minimized it, brushed it off, denied it, made fun of it, and stonewalled it. You did everything you could to avoid listening to or witnessing a friend's reality because their reality was yours, and it hurt like hell if someone named it, even if that someone was your devastated friend or partner, sitting in front of you.

Naming and sharing with words what happened to you is dangerous because it gives what happened a reality stamp. That is why silence sticks in collective trauma. You act as if your friend's experience wasn't a big deal because you will dwell on your own grief about what was done to you, and there is no time for grief in collective trauma.

You need to keep surviving, not grieving, and you need

to stay silent. There is a collective behavior of invalidating each other's experiences. When you are born into collective trauma, you are always invalidated. Everything that has happened to you is dismissed; you are deeply unseen, and your reality doesn't exist.

Each other's pain produces a deep sense of helplessness, and you fight it by not validating it. The bigger the dehumanization, the bigger the denial. Your container to tolerate injustice becomes wider and wider. It's a container of invalidation and your own non-existence.

You were assaulted because of your ethnicity, and everyone in your home was quiet or commented only with "good thing you weren't killed," and you continued with your day. You didn't hold onto that experience of terror or shock. You moved on as quickly as you could to the next thing you had to do.

You got pulled to the side and examined by the military because of your ethnicity? Well, it wasn't a big deal because you weren't killed.

You were denied space in a bomb shelter because of your ethnicity? Well, it wasn't a big deal, at least you survived.

The explosive detonated and demolished your home because of your ethnicity? Well, at least you weren't killed!

You had a rifle pointed at your chest and you begged for your life? Well, at least you weren't killed.

You stood in lines for food, were exiled and denied the identification card to become refugee, not citizen? Well, at least everyone had something to eat that night.

Your mother tried to commit suicide because she couldn't keep up? Well, at least she survived.

As soon as you dismiss the impact of what happened to you and others, you brace for the next even worse thing that could happen. In collective trauma, there is no end, no pause. It's all about brushing it off as quickly as you can, never talking about it, and bracing for another insult that will come any second.

That is the cycle of collective trauma for all who are living it. You keep denying, invalidating, and dismissing the horrific experiences of injustice done to you and your loved ones so often that you don't even know if what happened was real.

It felt as if you didn't actually live it. You don't know your own reality. You question yourself: *Did that really happen to me when everyone around me didn't see it?* You question if you are going crazy.

In collective denial, the collective trauma produces a collective craziness. Everyone feels crazy. What's ironic is that even if you talk about the impact of your experience and that you think you are going crazy, it will be brushed off. Everyone feels the collective craziness of collective trauma.

It's a soup of deeply isolated people who feel like they're going mad trying to survive, while not noticing they are boiling in a pot of collective pain.

INTERNALIZED OPPRESSOR

OPPRESSED FAMILIES KILL THE EXUBERANCE AND JOY in their kids. Not because they don't love them, but because they want to protect them, and the fear of violence gets stuck in their bones. That fear is passed down from their parents, grandparents, and ancestors.

If their child is strong, outspoken and vibrant, taking up space and living freely, it means they will be noticed, seen, condemned, taken away, and killed by their oppressor. An independent person is a threat to tyrants.

This traumatization and fear instilled in your parents or grandparents made them put you in a cage and tame your life force. They did this so you wouldn't be imprisoned, killed, enslaved, or forcibly sent to residential school by colonists and other entitled pricks.

They just wanted to protect you and didn't have the words or knowledge to explain to you why you could be harmed if you were allowed to be who you are. The cage that locked away your light came from a deep fear, love, and desire to protect you.

LET US DECIDE!

"WE DECIDE IF YOU GET TO BELONG!" SAID BRITISH colonists, while excluding ninety-nine percent of the people on this planet.

I guess we are now the ones who get to decide if they should belong to us—we, the commoners. All ninety-nine percent of us. Let me correct that, it's probably ninety-nine point nine-nine percent, since all those who do not come from noble lineage in Britain are considered hoi polloi.

WALKING ON MY KNEES SO I DON'T UPSET YOU

WHEN YOUR COUNTRY, YOUR COMMUNITY, YOUR neighbors, your school, and your colleagues repeatedly instill in you the belief that you are wrong—the wrong color, the wrong ethnicity, the wrong religion, or the wrong human—you withdraw into a life of isolation.

You believe your mere presence hurts those around you. They have made you believe that you are wrong, and that just showing up beside them will cause them discomfort and unease. You can feel it in the air, all the unspoken disdain of your presence.

The energy field shifts when you show up. You're not imagining it—that's your true experience because your nervous system is detecting threat cues. You're not making it up in your head. You can feel the shift when you show up.

Then you start feeling responsible for how you made them feel, and you just want to make it right and please them. You don't want them to feel any discomfort because of you, so you follow the subtle twitches in their faces and jump to serve at every smirk. You do all this to justify your presence.

In that kind of existence, an enormous amount of toxic shame is born inside of you. You believe you are a toxic human being. You cause other people to look at you with frowns on their faces, as if you entered the room smelling like rotten eggs.

Deep toxic shame sticks with you. It never goes away. It sticks to your bones, your arms, your legs, and it follows you until you stop taking any space in the world, including your office, your school, and your community, just to name a few. Toxic shame spreads to your kids, too.

It causes you to hide your essence. You dim your light because everyone around you has made you feel like you weren't wanted. Trust yourself; you're not making it up. Words or insults don't need to be spoken for you to know this.

It's a subliminal frequency, emanating from their eyes, their tone of voice, their micro-aggressive smirks, frowns, and sometimes from their casual comments about how you are less or wrong. They might say, "That immigrant!" as if you're not even a human.

Just read the word, *that*. That immigrant. That minority. That derelict. That female. That obese person. That disabled person. That queer person. That scum! That!

And what can you do but retract into the smallness of yourself in order not to hear those insults or upset anyone?

That's oppression. It is the loss of humanity inside of you. This shame you feel about yourself is what society, your country, your community, your neighbors, the media, and the government put on you. This shame is so deadly that it was one of the worst weapons I faced.

I had guns pointed at my forehead and chest more times than I care to remember, but this shame deprived me of my dignity and agency more than the guns. When you repeatedly have a gun pointed at your forehead, anger and righteousness show up, and you don't care if you are killed.

Some internal spite keeps you standing tall, but this continuous communal exclusion brings shame that destroys your dignity. It's in everyday moments that you see yourself as unwanted in society. This quality of shame is what is so deadly. This is what kills you, not the bullets.

Bullets would be less painful than constantly living with the feeling that you are worthless. The deep humiliation that you have no value because of your ethnicity, skin color, religion, choice of partner, or looks.

That indoctrinated shame, for me, was deadlier than any bullets. It left me on my knees, crawling for decades. For some, it impacts them for the rest of their lives.

WHAT'S IN ME
SCARES ME

LIVING A LIFE WITH INNER CONFLICT CREATED DUEL-ing forces inside of my body. One that wants to roar against injustice and say, "No more!" while the other part is too afraid, believing that if it rises from inside of my being, a dam will break loose.

The ensuing torrent will inundate people and places with the force of my suppressed anger that has been hidden for decades. That anger witnessed injustice and wants to swipe at those who caused harm. It wants to roar. It isn't really anger, but rather rage and revenge that swirl inside of me.

I see myself as a possible danger. Can the hurt one hurt? Can the terrified terrorize? Can the abused abuse? Can a beggar, pleading for their life, make others beg? Can the humiliated demand their dignity? Can those who were wronged, wrong others? Can the bearers of injustice claim their own justice?

The genocide I lived through still lives in me. I thought it could break a dam in me and kill many, as they had tried to kill me. Could it? I can still feel it. I am holding this force in me and I know I have to sit with this feeling for the rest of my life.

That force is in you, too. It can scare you. It's a byprod-uct of layered abuse. It is the thought that you might do the same as those who harmed you. It is a truth you feel inside of yourself when you survive horrific acts of violence and bloodshed. There is another force here, the terror that even if you roar, even if you let your voice be heard, you will end up alone, judged and ostracized. You will become even more isolated than you are now.

I live in a conflicted space. I want to roar for all the wrongs done to me and my people, and yet I silence myself to avoid being ostracized. I want to belong, and the cam that holds back the anger is so deep, it suffocates my screams. This is life spent in conflict. It is life with PTSD and trauma.

The conflict is just *there, inside of you*. This is what abuse does to you. You live in a space where you are scared you might harm others, and yet, you just want to belong.

WITHOUT YOUR PERMISSION, SIR, I MIGHT NOT LIVE

THE PURPOSE OF THE MILLENNIA-LONG PATRIAR-chy—if you're a woman—is to destroy all of your values, so all you have to hold onto is the beliefs of men. That is, the beliefs of entitled men, although some women wiggle their way in, too. They decide. They lead. They demand. They choose for you.

These men, typically older, wealthy men of self-pro-claimed authority and establishment, believe they are so important and precious that their values are the only ones to be accepted and followed.

You were born into this space. It was all that you and your parents knew, and you spent your life orbiting around the values of authority and privilege, obediently waiting for a man's permission and approval.

As an adult, you don't know what kind of permission it

is that you need, or where exactly it should come from; all you know is that it's definitely coming from somewhere above your head. That is the essence of living in a patriarchal system. It is the essence of the abuse of power. You are stuck, waiting for permission to live your own life, based on a man's belief of his privilege and entitlement.

Learn your rights and your own values. If you want to build and develop your own business, or marry someone you love, you don't need the permission of anyone who believes they are above you. No one but you can decide how you need to live your life.

You have a right to decide what you value, and to live life on your terms with no one's permission. Truth be told, you do not need permission to belong or be accepted, because in privileged eyes, you will never be equal. To them, you will always be someone who needs to follow, which is simply not true.

THEY TOOK HER SAFETY AWAY

SHE BUILT HER SAFETY AROUND HER BY MAKING friends all the time. She gathered her friends around her as a column of protective light. She built an escape. She built a fantasy land, a realm of joy. She somehow knew this was a way to escape when the harm of a man's hands arrived. In the hands of supportive friends, she was still able to fly.

When she was displaced, the safety she worked so hard

to build instantly erupted in the smoke of her detonating home. She disappeared from life and waited to be woken up in the supportive hands of her precious friends.

She knew what to do to make herself feel safe, but when she was left without her friends, over and over again, she resigned and let the man's hands do what they wanted. In her hurt, she just resigned.

POWER THROUGH

YOUR GRANDPARENTS, YOUR PARENTS, AND ALL OF your elders were proud of you when you powered through. You were probably praised and admired for it. It felt good to be capable and strong. What they didn't praise or culti-vate was the need to lean on others and receive help when you were vulnerable, fragile, tender, and tired.

I bet those states were not even recognized, named, acknowledged, or supported. If those states arose in you— or in them, they were quickly dismissed, minimized as a disruption, chalked up as weakness, even labeled as a plague. Those thoughts were simply not allowed in a trauma body, for the sake of survival.

If your ancestors were allowed to feel vulnerable, tender, and ask for help and support, they would be killed or left without the ability to work and feed their families. If your immigrant father said to his wife, "I just need to rest; I'm overwhelmed," he knew he wouldn't survive, and neither would his family.

This is passed down through generations. It causes you

to override your need to rest, and forces you to overachieve and overwork. There is always something else you need to power through.

If you wonder why you're always so exhausted, it's because it's stored in your bones. Your parents modeled how to power through, to never ask for help or even simply rest. For decades. For generations. This was passed down as some sort of legacy. Was leisure time ever allowed in your family or appreciated? No. Leisure was a privilege, not an option for survival.

I've witnessed so many people become terminally ill and keep this news a secret, feeling that they couldn't share their imminent death with anyone. They had to soldier through until their last breath, and of course not be a burden to anyone or be perceived as weak.

They powered through and died hiding their tenderness and need for help. They kept silent and they powered through until they died alone.

ONE PERSON HARMED YOU, SO SEVEN BILLION OTHERS DON'T STAND A CHANCE

WHEN TRAUMA AND NEGLECT HAPPEN IN OUR FAMILY of origin, the harm is usually done by one person. If we had the typical nuclear family of four, only one was the abuser, but the entire family unit felt unsafe for us as a child or a teen.

Having grown up in this kind of family, we're continuously scanning and sensing for any possibility that we might be harmed, as well as noting any resemblances to the person who hurt us when we were younger. Throughout our adult life, we keep detecting threats similar to our childhood abuser.

Any similarities to your father, or your mother, or your siblings can just pop up and you will be on high-alert. This detection method follows us to our social events, in our offices, and in our relationships. There are more than seven billion people on the planet, but the shadow of the one who harmed you will not leave you alone or give you a break. This prevents you from getting to know the rest of humanity and finding good people.

The image of our abuser is imprinted on our mind and body like our fingerprints on our fingertips. We miss so many good people in our lives while we are scanning and sniffing for one with a similar imprint.

Even when we meet good people and accept them into our lives, they come with a trauma-specific return policy, good for life. To use it, you just wait for the mask of kindness to drop and for their true face to appear. The face of the abuser. We can't let go.

COLLECTIVE TRAUMA

WITH COLLECTIVE TRAUMA, YOU FEEL AS IF THE entire world is against you, your family, your people, your ethnicity, and your skin color. If religion is present, your connection with your faith community may become tighter and your separation from the rest of the community greater.

Segregation is the outcome of collective trauma. It's what the oppressor wants because it makes it easier for them to have control over you. It's possible that you feel safe in that community. You get to be you. You don't feel othered. It's only you and your people.

You understand and can support each other, yet you isolate yourselves from the rest of humanity, depriving yourself of those connections and humanity of your light. You imprison yourselves, and that is what your oppressor wants. They want you to stay put and be tamed. You believe you have freedom of speech and some sense of support within your community, because your oppressors won't allow that freedom with them.

MY CLASS IS LESS

I had the wrong accent.

I was the wrong religion.

I was the wrong ethnicity.

I was the wrong class.

I became wrong the very moment that
I had the audacity to be born.

How dare I think I could have my own voice?

I consumed this awareness from everyone I stood behind.

You ask me why I cannot speak in front of others?

Ask yourself, were your values considered less?

Did the sight of your parents' car
provoke frowns on posh faces?

Did your hair smell of ethnic food from a Sunday BBQ?

Was your accent an insult to their Ivy League grammar?

Was your name too difficult to pronounce?

Was your loud tone considered rude?

You ask me why I cringe when people are around?

Come and stand behind my back.

I learned something along the way;
my accent is thick,
my grammar is shit,
the smell of kebabs perfumes my skin.

Come and stand behind my back.

My class is considered less,
and they can kiss my ass with their false pretense.

There is only fluff behind their composed
faces, patronizing tone, and Louis Vuitton.

When they see injustice, they are
scared for their own asses.

They aren't calling you to stand behind them;
it's not in them to stand up for someone who is less.

You, come stand behind my back.

Certainly, this is better than looking
at their condescending faces.

They want to scrub themselves clean
after just looking at our skin.

Come, stand behind my back.

Here, with me, your class will never be less.

You belong to the good, as you always should.

They are the ones who will always be behind,
so, stand tall and feel innate pride.

DIFFERENT SHADES
OF WHITE

I AM AN INVISIBLE MINORITY. I AM WHITE. I AM SCRU-tinized for being the wrong ethnicity. I was punished for having the wrong religion. I was dehumanized for my eth-nicity and faith, even though I wasn't aware of them as being mine. I didn't pray. I didn't know my identity until it was ter-rorized. I didn't understand until I faced persecution and spent years in exile.

I was systematically discriminated against and forced into poverty and homelessness. I am a child and adult of three wars. A child soldier. An army sniper. My chest and forehead were touched by the tips of rifles more than by kind human hands. So, I wonder where I belong. I am not a visible minority. Growing up in my home country, I was not seen as white in the privileged sense, and yet I am very white from the outside. Blue eyes. Blonde hair. Even now, as an immigrant, my whiteness is often othered.

I am one of the invisibles. I am othered. I am less. I wonder where the other invisible ones are, the ones who—like me— are seen as less. There must be thousands, perhaps millions of us. Each with different stories but the same invisibility and nowhere to belong.

MINORITY

No, take this away from me! It cannot be mine.

This dirt, this plague, this enclosure
of shame — it cannot be mine.

It's stuck to my skin and cannot be washed away.

It makes me revolt against myself. this
inherited religion and ethnicity of mine.

Hey, it is not mine! It is not mine!

I scream out loud, losing my friends, not
wanting to be in this skin of mine.

It feels like dirt. I have become someone
who no one wants to stand beside.

No one wants me around.

I am an unwanted smell, producing disgust in others' guts.

Take it away, take it away; it is not mine! Just take it away!

I am fed up with being ashamed of who I
am, of being despised by everyone else.

I want to be the same as you.

I want nothing of mine anyway! Just take it!

Take away everything that makes me less, and turn me into someone who is proper and right, someone who is decent enough for acceptance. Make me one of us!

I couldn't care less about what is
mine, just make me one of us!

I wail desperately, pleading to be accepted,
while giving away my essence.

This was inspired by feeling ashamed of my Serbian ethnicity in pre-war Croatia, and hearing my best friend's dad say no Serbs may enter his home, ever. I was left feeling wrong, washed in shame, deeply lonely, and ostracized by friends, the system, my country, and community. I dedicate this to all BIPOC, invisible minorities, and the people who were and are currently in war.

THE POSTURE OF THE OPPRESSED BODY

WHEN YOU COME FROM A LINEAGE OF OPPRESSION, the expectation of being invaded—of others taking over your body, your home, your land, your choices, your dignity, and your voice—is constant. There is no rest. You feel like, at any moment, someone is going to invade what is yours, what belongs to you, what is your birthright and human right. You feel as though you constantly need to defend those rights.

Living in this state is tremendously exhausting for the human organism. The body feels it like a load of heaviness in the bones, in the structure of the body's systems, in your muscles, in your fascia, and in your spine. That load of heaviness impacts your posture over time, causing it to either collapse or go into a rigid, armored position.

What is more important is that it becomes your normal state. You normalize this posture and might not even be aware of the heaviness of your body or how it carries trauma. That is the energy you emanate.

It isn't vital, sparkling energy that trauma states radiate. It's heaviness, alertness, cautiousness, tremored, or resigned energy. Look around or see yourself in the mirror when you are sitting or walking, or recall a memory of your parents and their posture.

Trauma bodies walk around burdened, and our posture mirrors our history. It tells our story. The body speaks of what we've endured without us telling our story.

In a collapsed posture, the shoulders go over the heart, the pressure of weight concentrates at the lower spine, the face is pulled down, the eyes look toward the ground, the front neck is withdrawn, and the chest collapses inward with a soggy, wet, heaviness in the long bones of the arms and legs. Trauma bends bodies over.

In rigid postures, your body is like a robot. Compact, braced, and constricted. The entire system is a block of cement.

The neck moves right and left in micro-rigid and sliced movements, the muscles of the face are taut and pulled up, the eyes move quickly, but the neck doesn't follow. The arms and legs are heavy and cold, and it looks like the limbs are disconnected from the torso. The demeanor of the body is one of heaviness and tiredness, but the eyes look hyperalert, as if they want to jump out of their sockets.

There are no light steps or effortless movements. Light and ease were taken away from our oppressed and traumatized bodies. There is no buoyancy or flow. The legacy of trauma is too heavy for our bones to carry.

I learned to acknowledge my burdened body. I am still alive, somehow. My body knew how to survive. For this, I love my body. Remember, your body is your homeland. It is your address throughout your life, and it can never be invaded or taken away from you.

It can be, and it was, dehumanized, but your body never left you. It is the most loyal part of you. Your bones can't be taken from you. What is written in your posture tells your legacy. Your ancestors sit in your bones. Your lived trauma sits in your bones.

When you acknowledge your disconnected body, your posture will change. Remember, your body is your altar. In it, honor the weighted legacy and stories your bones carry. That weight will turn into dignity and pride, and one day your posture will lift back up.

OVERLOOKED

I wish I was overlooked.
It would mean I don't matter, not even a tiny
bit. Not enough to be bothered with.

I wasn't overlooked.

In oppression and abuse you are never overlooked.
You are picked to be victimized, picked to be
played with, picked to be ostracized.

Yes, white skin, blue eyes, but the "wrong" ethnicity
and religion, which I never even knew I had
inside of me. I was picked so many times.
I was held at gunpoint more times
than I bothered to count.

I knew this religion of mine—and me, by
default—was so wrong and worthless
the first time a soldier's rifle caressed my
forehead, down to my right breast, crossing my
heart, touching another nipple and slowly going
up my chin and then back down my neck.

He did this in slow motion as if he was making his best art
piece, brushing the tip of my skin and painting a revenge
landscape fueled by deep, satisfying control over me.

He was aroused. I knew it. I could only look down.

Looking up meant I might die. He wanted
me to see the contempt on his face.
He was a god, and I was less.

In my periphery, I saw my father's white fingers
holding a bag. We tried to escape.

I was fifteen and my sister was eighteen.

I wish we were overlooked.
Maybe our dignity and the innocence of our youth
would have stayed untouched, somehow.

Maybe the wrongness and shame around myself and my
religion would not follow me throughout my entire life.

Maybe, if I had been overlooked. Maybe.

SO, I WAS GOOD?

So, I was good back then, but not now?
Compliant, submissive, voiceless, and obedient.
I *was* good, but I am not good now?
Hmm...I wonder why?

Is that fear in your eyes?
You look surprised, and yes, there is a
confused fear behind your eyes.
Are you sensing that you are losing
your sadistic power, somehow?
Yeah, I was good back then, but not now.
Something shifted, but you can't figure it out.

Ooh, does this discomfort you're feeling for
the first time make you lose ground
as the entitled, empowered, and
controlling abuser you are?
It disturbs you, but you still don't know how.

It is my voice and my oppressed power coming out!
Yes, I know I was good back then, but not now.
You still cannot figure out how?

I look taller. I am straightening my spine.
I am not looking down, but straight into your eyes.
You are sensing the demeanor of my protective anger.
I have come to life, that is why.

I am standing up for myself, and you feel threatened.

Yes, I know I was good back then, but not now.
So, you better run and hide.

199

THEY TOOK MY LAND AWAY

They shamed me for who I am and took my land away.

They moved me from my ancestral ground, as
if I were a toxin that spread around,
leaving only death behind.

They shamed my name and my
language, and looked offended,
as if hearing my name was an insult to their nice manners.

They came into my home and acted as if I was an
intrusive pest who didn't know how to behave,
as if I was the one who didn't belong—here, on my land.

They made me whisper and taught me to hide, to
leave my land and all my ancestors behind.

They took my birthright and blamed me
for the lineages I carry in my bones.

They shamed me for the descendants that I left behind,
when I was laid to rest with my own kind,
who they killed with contemptuous pride.

7

TRAUMA BODY

A TRAUMA BODY VERSUS A HEALTHY BODY

THE TRAUMA BODY CONSTANTLY CHASES LIFE FOR fear of being left out and missing the boat. A person without trauma, or someone with healed trauma, trusts life, people, and the choices coming to them.

It's chasing life versus having trust that opportunities are coming toward you. Fear vs. knowing. Antigravity vs. gravity. Braced vs. fluid. Hectic vs. calm. Never being good enough vs. having peace where you are at. A trauma body vs. a healthy body.

A healthy body will visit the states of a trauma body, but it will not get stuck there. The healthy body will feel it for a minute, or a couple of hours, or even a day, and then it will move back into a healthy, regulated state. That is its home base.

In contrast, the trauma body will remain stuck for years in states of chasing, fear, antigravity, bracing, and exhausting internal negotiation.

YOU LIVE IN A BRACED BODY

IN A TRAUMA STATE, ALL YOUR BODILY SYSTEMS— including your skeleton, muscles, diaphragm, fluid, and immune system—are compressed. The moment trauma happened, your systems braced, contracted, and constricted. Your entire being became rigid. The normal flow of blood and energy became abnormal.

There is no buoyancy in the trauma body, so your cells cannot be replenished or regenerated. This is the source of inflammation, a weakened immune system, chronic pain, and many illnesses. This is a trauma body.

When your nervous system doesn't get the chance to release and cycle through its trauma responses, you experience that compressed, braced, and constricted body for years, sometimes decades.

Notice how your abdomen is compressed, your diaphragm contracted, your chest braced, your neck tight on the side and back, and your eyes narrowed.

Your body can also respond to trauma by moving into a collapsed state, where you feel as if you are Jell-O, where there is nothing to hold you, and your arms and legs are disoriented, causing clumsiness and falling, both of which are common.

Interestingly, you probably haven't even noticed any of these symptoms, and yet you still know you experienced trauma. That absence of noticing is common for a trauma body. It is a disconnect from your bodily awareness. Braced and collapsed states become normal. You normalized them as the way your body is supposed to feel, and soon enough, the trauma body became the only one you remembered.

Maybe you didn't get to know the natural state of your chest or your pelvis in a toned, fluid, soft, and coherent way. How could you, when you lived a life filled with trauma? In a way, coherence can also happen in trauma patterns and dysregulated body states. Abnormal patterns get normalized.

In a healthy body, we want to see coherence and collaboration between the systems, with healthy containment and movement. For example, in the respiratory system, your breath is expansive, easy, and can move into your muscles and other systems without constriction. Your entire body is breathing and being fed with that breath.

In trauma, all the body's systems function in survival mode and are separated from each other, carrying loads of activations. The breath is shallow and rapid, not moving and feeding the other systems. Tissues are deprived of oxygen, the muscles are braced, your heart rhythm is in flux, your body temperature fluctuates, and more.

When you live for decades with PTSD and trauma, this is all your body knows, and so it makes this state coherent and normal in an unhealthy way. Your body is functioning by draining massive amounts of energy from you, and therefore has a shorter expiration date, meaning you will die sooner.

Being constricted, braced, or collapsed is your natural response to trauma, and you want to move your body out of this response while orienting toward safety.

You are stuck in a trauma response, and your body and mind are trying to sustain the enormous amount of life energy necessary to survive, while holding that braced and contracted state in every system of your body.

That is why you feel exhausted and drained, and you might not even know how it feels to be replenished and rested, because your body has normalized this trauma state.

WHY CAN'T I FEEL IT?

WE DON'T ALLOW OUR EMOTIONS AND SENSES TO rise up because we think they might overwhelm us so deeply that we will never be able to put ourselves together again. We think we will crumble into a thousand pieces, that it will feel like the moment when we fell apart, collapsed, and had a nervous breakdown; or we fear that we will be engulfed, shocked, and terrorized.

So, the brain subconsciously decides to shut down and disconnect, both from our feelings and from our bodies. It is a trauma response. *I will never feel any pain again*, we decide. We want to feel joy, but that's not how it works. We can't decide to only feel pleasant feelings.

We might decide the amount of time we spend with our feelings, but we cannot choose to only feel the pleasant ones and not the unpleasant ones, too. You either feel both or none. So as your brain decides not to feel because of the fear of what those feelings might remind you of, you stop living and go on autopilot.

You might wonder why you are never as happy or joyful as others. You might be perceived as artificial, dry, flat, numb, surface-level, shallow, slow, or disconnected. That is what trauma does to us. It makes us flat so we can survive and function in day-to-day life. You will dis-arm yourself to make sure you don't reach out to anyone and get hurt again.

You can spot a person with trauma on the street by just looking at their arms. They look as if their arms are separate from their torso, as if their arms are disembodied from their life. Those arms died a long time ago; they stopped reaching out.

Dis-armed, disembodied and disconnected, you become detached from your body, your feelings, yourself, and others.

Your body decided to disconnect from what you feel, so you never feel the anguish and pain you experienced back then. The fear of what you might feel is too overwhelming for your system.

To heal, you must start allowing yourself micro-feelings and micro-experiences in micro-moments. Just let that one micro-feeling in, then stop. Only one percent of a feeling, for fifteen seconds. That is a good start. The remote control is in your hands. You stop, you pause, and you rewind to experience it again if it feels yummy. If not, you fast forward.

You let micro-feelings in and notice how they feel, and notice that you are not falling apart. You are not overwhelmed, and you might be surprised to reconnect to your emotions and feel things about yourself and others again. Let those arms get attached to your body once more. One day you will be able to reach out to others and connect.

You are more than worthy of it. You are in charge of your feelings. Just make sure to always have support from kind friends, therapists, or the people around you, or, invite your ancestors, your soul people, your beloved animals, and your favorite oak tree. Create your support system. If there is too much in that micro-feeling to let in, your support system will be there to take it for you.

ARE YOU A SLOUCHER?

PROLONGED SHAME CAN PRODUCE A COLLAPSED posture in the trauma body.* The head hangs down, the neck is sunken, the shoulders collapse over the chest, the chest moves inward, the pelvic floor lacks tone, and the eyes look down in despair, not toward others.

I was told so many times by my parents to straighten my back. They seemed almost annoyed and kept asking me why I was always slouched. How ignorant of them to never realize that hidden trauma and shame lived inside of my slouched body. Why would they? Ignorance is bliss in traumatized families.

Look and observe. Move away from your phone and look at the people around you. We tell so many stories with our bodies. We tell stories of trauma, of gene mutations, of health woes. Notice, observe, help, make a connection, send a gentle gaze, and say a kind word. Say, "I care about you," when you look in the mirror, and you will stand taller day by day.

---

* According to the Centers for Disease Control and Prevention (CDC) common neural defects such as spina bifida impact an estimated 1,427 infants annually. Accordingly, it is important to note that not all curved spines are caused by trauma and disabled bodies are not inherently representative of trauma or shame.

WHY IS IT HARD TO LOOK INSIDE OF YOURSELF AND FEEL IT?

AN INDICATOR THAT YOU HAVE TRAUMA INSIDE OF you is that you are an expert at moving on to the next thing. You typically do this as soon as some deeper emotions or sensations become present inside of your body. You pick up your phone, you start talking too much, or begin nervously laughing, or you move on to the next relationship, the next venture, the next burning issue you need to resolve.

As long as the focus is outside of your body, it's fine. When that focus turns inward, it's anything but. Because think, what will happen if someone who has been victim- ized pauses in the moment of abuse and actually feels it? What will happen to the person who has just experienced an assault, insults, harassment, or neglect? How difficult would it be to fully feel a bodily experience?

If you paused and made space to become fully aware of that experience, an unbearable amount of turmoil, shame, abandonment, and pain would arise, and your heart would break. The most intelligent response, one that eases the pain of trauma, is to override all your feelings and bodily states in the moment of a traumatic experience.

It helps your brain to override your emotions and thoughts and redirect your attention toward what's outside of you, toward someone or something else so you don't feel what is happening inside of you. It can move you toward other people's problems, so you don't need to look at yours, and it creates self-deception, where you minimize and jus- tify things in order to be okay.

This protective response directs you to enter an altered state, where you are completely checked out: dissociation. That intelligent survival strategy stays with you for a long time, even years or decades after you've left an abusive environment or experience.

You keep overriding your feelings, but now that also includes overriding your state of joy and ease. The trauma brain dismisses all experiences in the body, not just the negative ones. That is why you cannot fully feel.

It's why you can't even defend yourself, because if someone was rude to you, you wouldn't allow yourself to register the experience. You can't feel your feelings and you definitely can't say something back like, "Don't talk to me that way."

You dismiss awkwardness and override it. You might even start talking to the person who's insulted you, like nothing happened. You dismiss it. You minimize it. That is self-abandonment, and it was the best strategy back then. In the moment of assault, the best response was to abandon yourself and not feel anything happening to you.

Now, you can learn to come back to yourself, learn to pause and feel. Learn to notice the present state inside of you, how it feels, and wait for an emotion to arise. It will not kill you, and it will not overwhelm you to the point that you will lose yourself.

Do it alongside your therapist or with someone else who is safe. Hold their hand and allow yourself to feel sorrow, exhaustion, fear, or even just that you are okay. Let that emotion be present and notice how it transforms into something else. Emotions flow, they move, and they change. Notice that.

It is a wonderful experience to know what your body is capable of. So, just pause and notice what happens for you, and sit with it. Nothing bad will happen after you notice your emotions or state. You will be fine. The threat is gone.

Nurture what comes up in your experience. It is yours.

Notice and name it out loud. Say, "I just experienced confusion. I just experienced curiosity. I just experienced anger."
Name it. Own it. It is yours. Do not override it, minimize it,
distract yourself with things outside of you, or rationalize it.

Own it, notice it, feel it, and let it move through you.
That is the path to embodying yourself and leaving behind
decades of self-abandonment in order to survive.

CAN YOU HUG EASILY?

ONE OF THE IMPLICIT RELATIONAL MOVEMENTS IS TO
reach. Reaching is an innate, subconscious movement. A
baby reaches out for a nipple to be fed, for the warmth of
their mom's skin, the comfort of holding a finger. A toddler
reaches out to be held and lifted up in the safe arms of a
parent when they're hurt. A child reaches out to safe hands
when they go down the slide, their arms reach out toward
those same, safe arms to be pulled up when they fall down.

It is a movement you might not even be aware of, until
you realize it is not fully developed in you. Are you reaching out to people without even thinking and questioning it,
or are you assessing if it's okay to reach out? Do your arms
even reach out at all? What is the level of movement from
your arms toward people who are close to you?

As a child, did you have safe hands there to meet you,
hold you, and lift you up when you reached out for support?
Were your hands met with the safe hands of others?

Do you have those free, uninhibited movements toward
people, or is there an unexplainable wall of constriction

between you and others? What holds you back from reaching out? Typically, it is relational trauma and an unsafe environment during childhood, even if you had a parent who you loved.

It was just not safe for you to reach out, or it was an environment of neglect, where your parents or caregivers were too busy, or absent, or judgmental. Perhaps you had a mother who felt anxious and unsettled, so you couldn't reach out when you needed her. Maybe you were slapped or shamed when you reached out for something you wanted.

Now—as an adult—the free, uninhibited relational movement of reaching out doesn't happen for you. Notice other adults around you who can't reach out, or even initiate reaching out. It's deeply saddening and such a lonely, conditioned response to have.

Look at the arms of those adults. They look flat and pushed down. Trauma arms always look disembodied and dis-armed. Are you dis-armed?

When you are dis-armed, you can't reach out for a hug or to be held, because of the imprint of neglect and abuse growing up. Notice your arms and let them slowly move up and out toward someone who feels safe. You can start by hugging a tree, or reaching out to your dog. Allow your arms to spontaneously reach out and hug someone or something you love.

Notice if you are cemented and unable to move when you want to hug them. Do you feel awkward and uncomfortable? Think about who was dis-armed in your family. Who simply couldn't hug? Arms tell so many trauma stories.

Observe, listen, and reflect on what stories you hold in your bones, and love your body. Love yourself. Start and finish your day with your arms in a self-hug. Let someone just hold you in their arms, once you reach out to them.

WHAT KEEPS YOU EXHAUSTED?

IN TRAUMA, THE BODY IS ALWAYS HOLDING YOU IN ONE of two states. One is braced, and the other is collapsed. When you are in a braced state, you are hyperalert, easily startled, hypervigilant, and your entire organism is compressed.

Throughout time, your body will simply not have the energy to sustain a braced state. There is an enormous amount of minute-to-minute energy needed to keep you in that survival response. When help and release don't come, the body's only option is to abruptly drop into a collapsed state.

In that place, there is no energy left, no muscle tone, and your entire system feels wobbly. It's a place of despair and resignation. Moving into one of those two states, braced or collapsed, is a normal trauma response, but it is not normal to be stuck in either of those states for years. Unfortunately, many people with trauma spend their lives between those two states.

You can be hypervigilant, going nonstop like a hamster on the wheel, and then you just crash down and are too tired to get out of bed. What you want to do with your trauma therapist is build your nervous system's capacity to move in and out of those states, and find a place of regu ation and safety—your ventral place.

A ventral place is where you feel safe in your body, safe with others, and where you are able to engage, be creative, do self-care, and seek support. Though a ventral place is unfamiliar territory to you, it is a place that already exists inside your system. It is accessible, and with the right therapy and support, you will move out of those two exhausting extremes and finally allow your body time to rest, rejuvenate, and replenish.

WORDS DON'T TELL
YOUR HISTORY

OBSERVE YOUR BODY. HOW DOES IT SPEAK? WHAT STO-
ries do your muscles express? How does your muscular system
write the history of your internal state? How do you move your
pelvis and long bones? Are your hips leading, or your head?

All your emotions are communicated through your bodily
movements. The way you express your micro – and macro-
movements tells your trauma history. The movement of your
body is an expression of your relationship with the environment around you and your internal processing of it.

You do not need to talk. Observant eyes will notice a flu-
idity, flow, silkiness, and juiciness in your movements, or
they'll see cut-down, compressed, braced, rigid, dry, stiff,
and startled movements. The regulated body is a river; the
trauma body is a robot. The body is writing a story of your
past, and movement is the book of your trauma history.

WHAT DOES THE BODY NEED FROM THE MIND?

IS THERE COMMUNICATION COMING FROM YOUR BODY to your mind? Or is the mind only communicating with your body? Who has the mic all the time? Your body or your mind? Is there even the possibility of listening to what the body needs from the mind?

Have you ever asked yourself what the body needs from the mind? Is it to soften, quiet down, see your body, and take a step back? What exactly does the body need? If the body can talk, it will ask the mind to quiet down. It will ask the mind to stop judging, over-expecting, over-demanding, and shaming. Often, though, the trauma body can't talk. Or, the trauma mind doesn't hear what it is saying.

If the trauma body could speak to the mind, it would say:

Can you honor me? Can you see me? Can you stop ignoring me? Can you stop punishing me? Can you stop abandoning me? I feel like an abused child, hurt by a neglectful loved one. This is what you are doing to me, neglecting me as if I am that child, left without support, unseen and cut off from the rest.

I feel as if I don't belong to you, as if I am a burden. It feels like the abuse and neglect you know so well. This is what you are doing to me, to your body. I am a boat, and I cannot use my engine if you are driving me against the current. I will die of effort, and yet you cannot acknowledge me. Can't you see if I die, you will die too?

BREATHE IN SELF

THE TRAUMA STATE RESTRICTS YOUR BREATH. WHEN you are in danger, you do not breathe fully. The survival brain stops your breathing so the perpetrator cannot hear you. For many, the body still lives in trauma, and you can detect it by the constriction of breath.

The trauma body believes — on a subliminal level — that there is still some ongoing danger, even though the threat left years ago. Notice when you last exhaled in full safety, when you last softened your shoulders and the back of your neck. Can your body finally breathe?

CAN THE OPPRESSED REST?

BEING VULNERABLE IS NEVER ALLOWED IN oppressed families. It is like we are genetically incapable of noticing the need to be nurtured, nourished, touched, comforted, and taken care of. Having that need would mean taking a rest and being vulnerable. It would mean you need to pause and have downtime.

How could you pause and rest when you constantly had to survive and fight to save your life? How could you allow yourself to rest when, for your and your family members' entire lives, you have been refugees, displaced, immigrants, farm workers, enslaved, overpowered, robbed, exiled, and dehumanized? The body cannot rest. It needs to survive.

A SHORT TRAUMA HISTORY

Trauma in the body can be summed up as
bracing, numbing, and collapsing.

ARE YOU VIBRATING ON A TRAUMA FREQUENCY?

RECORD YOUR VOICE AND LISTEN TO IT. CAN YOU
hear a recording of your voice without cringing? How quickly
do you want to remove yourself from that experience? Does
it make you uneasy? Do you want to jump out of your skin?

If you wonder why you can't stand to hear a recording
of your voice, it's because you are listening to the vibration
and frequency of your internal trauma. Your whole body is
receiving resonance, the vibrational tone of your painful,
traumatic experiences through your vocal cords. It is bounc-
ing back into your nervous system.

How you resonate with the frequency of your tone is a
clue to your inner state. The tone indicates so much. The
subtle frequency. Listen around you—whose vocal vibra-
tions seem off? Who has strained, constricted, and braced
vocal cords? Whose voice gives you unease or even anxiety?

It can feel like someone's tone of voice is penetrating your skin and invading your space.

If someone denies they have trauma, ask them to listen to a recording of their voice and let them observe how their nervous system responds to it. Do they move toward safety and playfulness, or toward restlessness, cringing, and fidgeting? Our vocal cords translate our internal state of safety, suppressed memories, hidden traumas, and pain; they vibrate at a trauma frequency.

TOLERATE

HOW CAN YOU LEARN TO TOLERATE YOURSELF WHEN you were not tolerated growing up, or when your own parents could barely tolerate you? All of your actions, feelings, states of being as a child were that you were too much, too disturbing to witness, see, or handle, and your parents and other adults were forced to tolerate you when you showed up.

Do you have to tolerate yourself as an adult now, too? It's as if—as a child—the energy coming from you was *so* big and *so* damaging, that it overwhelmed your parents every single time. It was as if they witnessed Godzilla come out of you whenever your dad was just about to watch a game on TV, or read a magazine.

Or like some monster inside of you was about to ruin the planet by singing and dancing in the family room when mommy just wanted to have her glass of wine. When you grow up in a family where your parents only tolerated you, it makes you feel like everything about you, and everything you feel inside, is too much.

You become ashamed of what comes up for you, as if everything that you feel is wrong, as if on a fundamental level, you are wrong. Any emotions are too much, too excessive, too overwhelming, and definitely shouldn't be seen, because now — as an adult — your partner or friend would then have to tolerate you.

Feeling angry is too much, feeling joyful is too much, and feeling happy is too much. You don't even know what is okay to feel and to what extent you can feel it. The body remembers and warns against expressing any emotion that was perceived as too much when you were a child, any emotion that caused someone else to have to tolerate it, to tolerate you.

In this way, you learn to hide what is happening inside of you from everyone, and you learn to minimize it. Every state of being. You become flat, turning into someone who doesn't have any specific likes, dislikes, or wants. Your value system is undefined, and you go along with whatever.

You wonder why you cannot express joyfulness and happiness out loud, or even feel it? Because it wasn't tolerated in your family, and neither were your needs and wishes. So, you shut it all down.

You learned to not tolerate anything that could be slightly overwhelming for your body. Your body cannot fail you, your body cannot get tired or sick, because you will not tolerate it. The mind judges the body. The body is not allowed to be too loud.

When you had all that energy and were singing as a child, you were too loud and too much, so your body learned to quiet all its vibrant energy in response. Now, when you feel panic coming up in your chest, it feels like too much, too loud, and you can't tolerate anything that comes up from you.

You fear it, you judge it, you criticize it, and you run away from it. The same way your parents did. It is excruciating how we continue our parents' work of punishing ourselves because we were not tolerated.

What you need to cultivate is an enormous amount of compassion for yourself. You can envision yourself as the mother you never had, as someone who can hug you, and be with your fears, and your exuberance, and your aliveness, and your muchness as long as you need them.

When all these states show up inside of your body, do something new. Embrace them. Don't dismiss or judge them. That is what your parents did, so do the opposite, in spite of them if that makes it easier for you. Whatever works for you and the beautiful muchness of your younger self.

THE BODY REMEMBERS

DO YOU WONDER WHY YOU ARE REPEATING THE SAME pattern over and over again? You do this because trauma remembers the first time a painful experience occurred, and now, your survival brain and your nervous system react to similar experiences in the same way, just like they did the first time.

Even if you are an adult, the trauma brain will catapult you into the same freeze response you had as a five-year-old. You will become silent, numb, and unable to move. Your body remembers and responds the way it did the first time.

EXHAUSTION

TO RESTORE MY BODY FROM SURVIVAL EXHAUSTION, it will take at least three lifetimes of complete solitude and peace.

WERE YOU RIDICULED?

WHEN SOMEONE SHAMED AND RIDICULED YOU, IT left a vast emotional wounding that shows on your face. Showing expressions of fear, nervousness, or joy on your face signals abusive people to attack and ridicule you even more. Your survival strategy—in order to protect yourself from being shamed—was to develop a flat affect and stop expressing any emotions.

You became a facade of yourself, a concrete wall, so predators couldn't recognize anything happening inside of you. The entirety of your outside became still.

Notice children in school, for example. Observe who's calm and still. Stillness is a survival strategy. Unfortunately, schools are largely not trauma-informed, leaving many students who demonstrate loud and clear signs of abuse unnoticed by their teachers and school systems. For a long time, I only displayed six or seven basic expressions out of the ten thousand available to a human being.

I used around four or five facial muscles out of the forty-three available. Just look at those numbers. This is what being shamed did to me and what it has done to so many other trauma survivors. It deprives us of expressions, it freezes our ability to show the life inside of ourselves.

Pay attention and notice how many expressions and muscles you're actually using. Are you hiding yourself, or freely showing what's happening on your face? You might recognize how the unsafe environment you lived in made you camouflage your face with stillness.

From the outside, it can be perceived as if you lack emotions or empathy, but the truth is, you feel immensely; you just learned to protect yourself from terror.

On the opposite end, someone can develop the habit of expressing so-called easier emotions to hide their more painful ones. This can lead to people being described as fake or "too happy." They can express a menu of socially acceptable expressions, not their true feelings, in order to avoid their trauma. Their face will translate this protective deception by actively expressing what they consider safe emotions, as long as none are connected to their inner suffering, or reveal that they are frightened or unconfident.

Here's an exercise to help you recover your facial expressions. Touch your face with the tips of your fingers. Feel your face and the forty-three muscles within it. Welcome them back. Let your muscles soften from the inside out.

You can relax at home and play with as many expressions as you want. Welcome them back. If you are someone who expresses happiness or other safe emotions in order to hide your pain, then let your face settle, pause, and rest.

Whoever did this to you doesn't own the rights to your liveliness, vitality, or life force. Let your face show all that you've suppressed. Allow your facial muscles to paint the landscape of your inner life and show the world the richness you have inside.

HOLD YOUR TONGUE

THE PAIN IN YOUR JAW AND GRINDING OF YOUR TEETH comes from unexpressed anger. Did you have to hold your tongue? Did you witness your mother holdirg her tongue? Were you allowed to speak up, to say no, to scream, to call for help, to call for justice, or did you hold your tongue? Were you loyal to your family by saying nothing?

An enormous amount of survival anger is stored in your caged mouth. Suppressed, braced, protective anger sits in your jaw for decades. At the same time you're holding your mouth back, your pelvis is holding back, too. The pelvis and jaw have almost the same anatomy.

If you have been assaulted, your pelvis and your jaw will respond simultaneously in a braced, tight, protective response. Those body parts will keep the memory of that holding, and will feel unsafe letting go.

This is a form of trauma held in your body. Years of hold-ing in survival states causes a lack of tone and a lack of oxygen coming into the system. This means your cells aren't replenished and rejuvenated within your muscles, there is no radiance or color in your face, and no awareness of your pelvic floor. Due to this lack of cell regenera-tion, inflammation, TMJ pain, migraines, gum issues, and even endometriosis become common symptoms of the trauma body.

Think of how many times we had to hold our tongues, even in the midst of an assault, because we didn't want to embarrass our family name or cause a fuss n the commu-nity. This pain in our jaws and pelvis didn't start with us. It started with our mothers and grandmothers. They, too, knew how to hold their tongues in order to survive.

IF OUR ORGANS AND BODIES COULD SPEAK

WHAT WOULD OUR ORGANS SAY IF THEY COULD speak? Have you ever wondered? What would your bones, your muscles, and your body parts say? The mind always speaks—it never stops—it's always analyzing, demanding, and planning. But what would your organs say when it comes to telling your trauma story?

My stomach would say:

I can't function when I don't feel supported and have social safety around me. My entire digestive system hurts because of our fear of rejection. I will stop accepting food when I don't feel safe. I can't digest food while we're sitting by someone who makes me feel uneasy and unsafe. Every time we have to socialize, I am in pain or nauseous. Please, sit near kind people who make us feel safe.

My intestines would call out and say, "Protect me, protect me!" But, when that protection doesn't come, my intestines cannot be at ease. So, they get louder. "No one heard me," they say, "but I won't give up. Maybe I need to exaggerate or make a scene in order to tell you what I need. My only options are to become explosive or completely shut down." (Does this remind you of your IBS?)

The trauma liver is stuck in the past, going over memories. It is too scared to even think, much less speak, about the future. It needs to feel the inner self. The liver wants to discover your inner needs, your wishes, and the creativity you were never allowed to have.

Without a sense of self, the body has no drive. Lethargy and pessimism are all that's left in the liver, "What's the point?"

it asks. "I don't matter anyway, and I can't fix what's wrong." What it actually wants is for you to discover who you are.

Your brain stem in the back of your neck is wounded by your overthinking of every single detail, making sure you are not late, replaying your fears — like your fear of flying and your fear of forgetting something — or overplanning everything because of your constant fear of what might go wrong. The brain stem — the central place of PTSD — is silent, too tired to talk. But, it wants certainty and despises change and uncertainty. So, love your brain stem and tell it that you will be there for all unknowns.

Your kidneys are speaking too. They say, "I am so alone. I cannot always be self-reliant and push forward; I need to lean on others." The place of deepest loneliness is in your kidneys. If they could speak, they would say, "Please lean on someone so I can rest."

The pelvis speaks of a lack of fundamenta protection. It speaks about how it has fought throughout your life, and still can't regain awareness. The pelvis is stiff. It screams about surviving and fighting for life. The pelvis is the place of your deepest fear. If the pelvis could speak, it would say, "Don't live in shame for staying frozen and believing you betrayed me. We will learn when we need to say no and seek support."

The heart is begging for connection and belonging. It wants to land in the safety of someone's arms. If the heart could speak, it would say, "Support me from the back and protect me from the front. With your hands and loving eyes, please connect to others."

If your lungs could speak, they would wail. They would mourn and cry out over your lost innocence and love.

If your throat could speak, it would roar and take up space. It would uncage your silence and let go of the burden of family loyalty.

If your shoulders and torso could speak, they would say, "I have been clenched down for a long time. I want my dignity back!" If you were to unclench them, then they would lift up.

If your skin could speak, it would say, "I am tired of absorbing wounds and shame. It is time to move away."

If your eyes could speak, they would say, "I am done with looking at the ground. I want to look up and connect with people who are kind."

What would your organs say if you could listen to them?

BACK-TO-BACK

WHEN YOU CLOSE THE FRONT OF YOUR HEART TO people who have never-ending requests and demands, your back becomes stronger and wider. Your body intuitively welcomes dignity into your spine, where it belongs.

ORGASM

ORGASM IS A SPACE OF SURRENDER AND EXPANSION. Only ten percent of women can reach climax during intercourse. If you wonder why it is so challenging for you, think about what your body needs to do to get to that place. It needs to surrender into the hands and body of another human who is completely safe and consistent, allowing your nervous system to relax.

What the brain remembers about surrender and expansion is different. Did you grow up in a place of safety or a place of constant uncertainty? Were any of your relationships totally safe? Did you have adults or partners around you who you could surrender to and share anything that was happening to you?

As a child, were you able to run to your mother's arms, or toward your sibling or dad, and cry your heart out? Or did you have to withhold because your body didn't feel safe?

Were you allowed to go to your family members or to school with full enthusiasm and exuberance, wanting to share your excitement, your ideas, and your talents? Or did they cut you off, and maybe even laugh, dismiss, or shame you?

At that moment, your body got stuck and made a memory imprint of this. It remembers, *When I feel expansive and joyful, I'll be shamed and unsafe.* Your body — in order to subconsciously protect you — began preventing any expansion or surrender inside of you.

There is something that kicks in and cuts off your pleasure when you approach feeling anything enjoyable. That something is trauma, which has conflated expansion with shame. The body remembers.

The body knows that when you surrender with joy and exuberance, people reject or ridicule you, causing another wave of shame. That is an imprint of what happened, and why you cannot orgasm or be uninhibited during sex.

The body holds this conflated memory. Every time you approach expansion and surrender, your body inhibits and prevents it because it doesn't want you to ever feel the shame you did back then.

Sit with this. Recall what happened in the past. Who shamed you when you were about to surrender your joy and excitement to them? It can be as simple as sharing a picture you were really proud of and having someone mock it. That is an imprint in your brain.

When it comes to your partner, notice if they are truly safe for you. Is your partner someone who makes toxic comments, or who you just can't fully trust? Or are they someone who is truly genuine and loving? Share this chapter with them. Let them know why and how your body is responding to past trauma. In a safe space with a sex therapist, as well as on your own, explore micro-moments of surrender in the safe hands of others, with full consent.

WHY YOU CAN'T
MAKE ME COME

You got upset because I wasn't coming.

You put in so much effort and spent your precious money.

You were penetrating me to prove yourself.

Once again you were the star of the
night, in your own eyes.

My not coming dimmed your shine.

You couldn't understand why your hard work—you were
dripping with sweat—did not make you an alpha.

You had to sit on the throne so you could gloat.

The harder you tried, the more you tasted failure.
It was a reminder of where you grew up.

The further I was from coming, the more your
mind yelled that you were failing again.

You projected your inner disgust onto me, making
me the culprit of your low self-esteem.

In your narcissistic mind, you left me dry.

In your presence, my body could not surrender.

Remembering the insults you'd flung, my
body didn't trust itself to come.

Your unsafe presence was keeping me cut off from
innate expansion and orgasmic surrender.

ARE YOU A HEADLESS CHICKEN?

EMOTIONAL EXPERIENCES ARE STORED INSIDE OF YOUR body's systems—your skeletal system, muscular system, nervous system, fluid system, viscera system, and endocrine system. Memories of trauma live in one or more of your systems. Trauma has an imprint, a memory, a scar, and a pattern.

The mind interprets and applies meaning and words to the trauma that your body holds. Your organs will not use words to express your states, needs, and memories, but they will use the senses.

When there is attunement and friendship between your mind and body, the mind will start decoding the organs' language and begin describing your bodily sensations and stored body memories with words. This is what we teach clients in somatic therapy. We are building unity between their mind and body.

In trauma, many people are detached from what is happening below their heads. It's as if nothing exists down below, or what does exist is solely an annoyance. Certainly, Western medicine has encouraged this belief and split the body and mind centuries ago.

The mind becomes something that psychotherapists work on, and the body is the domain of physicians. You go to a doctor without your head, like a headless chicken, and to your therapist with only your head—as if you were decapitated—leaving the rest of your body at home.

Take a moment with these questions. When I ask if your mind is aware of your body, what comes up for you? How does your mind feel toward your body? Is it dismissive, judgmental, or annoyed? Does your mind want to see your body? Will it tend to it? Does your mind obsess over and only listen to the negatives, like the body's cues of sickness? Is your body a place of fear your mind runs away from? Is your mind tired of anticipating the first signals of a panic attack from your body? How unfriendly is your mind toward your body?

And how does your body feel about your mind? Take a moment here. Is your body scared of your mind?

Has it been routinely dismissed by your mind, so it can't give an answer? Is your body scared of your mind's judgment and condescension? Is your body fully present and confident while taking space? What do you feel? How old does your body feel? What is your body's state? Is it like a child, waiting for the mind to make a decision and a plan, without consulting the body?

How old does your mind feel? Does it feel like a critical parent? Pause and observe. Between your mind and your body, who is the child and who is the parent? Does your body feel neglected by your mind, as you felt neglected by your parents growing up?

Is your body unseen, and unheard, with no right to exist, to take up space, to be cherished and celebrated, to make a choice and decide, as you were when you were a child? Is your body a reflection of you when you were a neglected child? Is your mind your perpetrator? Is your mind abandoning you? Take a moment and notice. Observe the split between your body and mind.

What is true is that your body and mind are a unit. If you didn't have trauma, your body would lead and your mind would follow. They would dance in shared knowing, and lean on one another. They would be two loyal companions and friends. If this hasn't happened yet, that's okay; it is beginning to happen right now as you read this.

You just need to move toward a place of awareness of this split and the possibility of reuniting, holding, nurturing, loving, trusting, and befriending. That is where you need to go—to home base, the home of your body, the unity of mind and body. This can be your best journey yet.

Let your body and mind get to know each other; and don't allow them to reject and abandon each other the way others once rejected and abandoned you. Let them nourish each other, and let your body be seen, celebrated, and nurtured. Let your body know that it matters to you, to your mind, and to your soul.

Tell your body all the things you didn't hear when you were neglected and abused. Let your body know, and notice how your mind will cry over your body with love and care. This will be your homecoming.

IMPULSE

THE IMPULSE TO SIMULTANEOUSLY HELP OTHERS AND abandon your personal needs runs through your trauma body. It overrides your energy levels and overestimates your ability to help.

It forces you to betray yourself by always being there for others, when you can't even be there for yourself. It's a silent killer and an unexplainable force coiled in one.

RESPONSIBLE
FOR OTHERS

TRAUMA CAN CREATE AN ENORMOUS AMOUNT OF responsibility and accountability for others You know you were victimized, and yet when you share your experiences, you feel the need to manage the feelings and discomfort of others.

You dismiss what happened to you, as if your need for support doesn't matter, as if you weren't the one who was abused. Your focus is on how other people feel about your story, and that responsibility causes you to ignore your own emotional state and needs.

You shut down your voice, and your truth remains silenced. This is what happens in a victimized and blamed mind, which develops through mistreatment and trauma. The trauma fog makes you feel responsible for other people's emotions all the time, even when you aren't doing anything wrong.

Your abuser made you responsible for their behavior and emotions, and now, when you attempt to share your memories, you feel the same nagging sense of accountability for how others will respond to your story. This is trauma.

This is why generational trauma exists, and why we never speak about our abuse. It's not because we lack support, but because of the responsibility we take for the discomfort of those around us. This constant responsibility for the feelings of others is a burden of the trauma mind.

In my therapy practice, I've often witnessed clients minimizing their stories due to their concern for how I feel, and whether or not I have the capacity to help them. Even though they are paying a trained professional to help them with their PTSD and trauma recovery, they hold themselves and their stories back because of this misguided sense of responsibility.

HOW SHAME SPEAKS

SHAME PROTECTS YOU FROM FEELING MORE SHAME by giving you disapproving thoughts like, *I have to, I should, I must,* and *I better.* Shame never encourages you with thoughts such as, *I can, it's okay not to, I can learn,* and *I only have to do what feels right for me.*

Can shame pause and recognize that you can protect yourself, before it jumps to self-judgment? Can you tell your shame that you are learning to speak for yourself and to say no? Can your shame understand that you are learning boundaries and that you are in a safe space now? Yes. Once shame witnesses how you are keeping yourself safe and protected, it will stop exhausting you.

STOP ASSUMING

DON'T ASSUME PEOPLE WILL DO THE SAME FOR YOU as you have done for them. Don't assume that if you take time out of your busy schedule to do something for someone else, they will reciprocate. Don't assume that they will see your needs the way you see theirs. Don't assume that they will jump to take care of you the way you have for them. It won't happen. You need to recognize your own needs, acknowledge you are deserving of help, and ask them to help you.

However, understand that people have the right to accept your request, refuse it, or even stay undecided. They may even become defensive. That's okay. This is how you claim your space, claim your existence, and learn you matter.

This is how you stand up for yourself, how you self-advo-cate and stop self-abandoning. Every time you stay quiet and don't express your needs, you abandon yourself. You might assume people will see you in need and come to your rescue, but this keeps you a victim your entire life. It leaves you waiting for a parent or a prince to come and save you.

This is common with adults who have developmental trauma. You don't learn how to communicate your needs, and you might not even know what your needs are in the first place. Placing unspoken expectations on others to meet your needs is a sign of emotional immaturity, regard-less of your age.

Worse, it leaves you with deep resentment toward yourself and the world around you. Growing up, you were probably harmed, ridiculed, dismissed, or rejected if you expressed any needs. That is the core of trauma and the reason you've remained silent. Expressing your needs wasn't an option for you.

As you learn to express your needs, you also need to learn to say no to others. Just as others have the right to say no to you, you have the right to do the same. That's normal and healthy.

Blaming, punishing, or ridiculing someone who is expressing their needs is abuse, like you experienced in the past. Saying no, or taking time to decide if you want to help is your right, and your decision needs to be respected. But do not assume people will recognize your unspoken needs.

8

STILL, YET
POSSIBLE

HOW DID I RISE?

How did I rise and raise myself?

With the backbone of my painful past.

With the many lifetimes and ancient wisdom in my spine.

EMBARRASSED BY YOUR OWN VULNERABILITY

DO YOU FEEL EMBARRASSED HAVING ANOTHER person sit with you when you feel vulnerable or tender, or when you are in pain? It's almost surprising to have someone willing to be with us in our painful moments. It reveals how rarely we had a companion during times of heartbreak and distress. Maybe a pet was there, but never another person.

It feels strange. It's awkward to have a human soul beside

us in our tender human moments. By default, the dominant part of the trauma mind wants to shut the world out and revert into a self-reliant state where we self-soothe, licking our wounds on our own, because we don't want to burden anyone.

But maybe you can listen to another part of your brain, the part that knows your body and soul are longing to be taken care of and comforted by a soothing voice and the safe presence of someone who wants to sit beside us.

Maybe, finally, you can receive support for the experiences you are going through, and realize that you are not a burden. Someone genuinely wants to help you. That is worth feeling awkward and embarrassed.

LIGHT IN YOU

How brilliant and valuable you are!

Remind yourself of who you are.
I know you are dismissing my words right now.
That is what neglect and abuse does to us.

See your friends, see how they shine when you show up.
See yourself in the mirror
and remind yourself of who you have become.
No, do not run away. Truly see your kind eyes,
your divine essence.

See what someone robbed from you.
See your beauty, which they couldn't stand to see.

See your light, which couldn't shine over the
darkness of their pettiness and crime.
Your light was a reminder of the
darkness they carried inside.

See that light again, and remind
yourself who you have become.
What you see is your inner brilliance shining so bright.
Remind yourself, don't look down.
You are strong enough to witness your own light.

Let me hold your hand, and let's look up.
Your eyes are longing to see your inner spark.
Remind yourself of who you have become.
It is divine love and pure beauty,
the beauty of your center, that still lives inside.

Do not hide; let's look up and meet
yourself after all this time.

BADASS

THE MOMENT WILL COME WHEN YOU SHIFT FROM
how the world perceives you, to how you perceive the world.
How *you* perceive the world. Yes, you.

You get to have an opinion about others! That is the
moment when you encompass your adult body and adult
mind. It is a moment when you become a badass. Welcome
yourself!

IS THIS NORMAL?

BECOMING NORMAL STARTS WHEN YOU RECOGNIZE that you have the right to make a choice. Very few people with trauma know what it is like to have a choice. It was never an option, not even a possibility. You were never taught that you were allowed to say yes or no, or that you changed your mind.

The conditioned mind goes along and puts up with other people's opinions and choices for decades. You continuously put up with things that you don't even like. It doesn't have to be abuse. These things can be insidious and benign, but they put you in a position to compromise and go along with something you don't want for yourself in the first place. Just another helping of requests for you to load onto your plate because of subtle blaming and guilting your receive. Nothing big and direct but just a drop of conditioning on your heart.

Subserviently, you compromise all of your wants for other people's wants. You don't even think you have a choice to opt-out. It's autopilot living, day by day, year by year. You normalize it, and compromise becomes your life. You simply put up with it. This isn't normal.

You disappear, lose your integrity, lose your honesty with yourself and others. You no longer know who you are, what your true limits lie, and what your capacity is. You even lose your own needs, forgetting something as basic as what it is that you want.

When you see yourself as a human being with a basic right to accept, decline, allow, and decide what you can and can't do, what you do and don't want, you will no longer ask if this is normal. It will feel normal. It will feel right.

You have a choice to decide what is done to you and your life. That is normal. You don't have to go along with everyone else's needs and preferences and become complicit in the disappearance of who you truly are.

CURIOSITY

CURIOSITY IS EXPRESSED DIFFERENTLY IN TRAUMA bodies. Curiosity requires engagement, the flow of ideas, and connection. It requires you to move forward, to the outside, toward others, and into the world. In trauma, the entire body is shut down and remembers that engagement caused actual harm and trauma.

It doesn't mean curiosity doesn't exist—it does—but it will never be expressed with others while trauma is alive in the body. The way that innate curiosity gets expressed is through imagination—a gift of dissociation from trauma—and from there, poets, writers, artists, storytellers, and musicians are born.

Curiosity lives in trauma minds and engages in the realms of pure flow and connection with the divine, not in the world of people that surrounds us.

WHAT I NEED
FOR HEALING

Don't judge me.

Don't defend yourself.

Don't blame me.

Don't blame yourself.

Don't leave.

Do not try to use humor to minimize it.

Look at my eyes.

See me when I share my experience.

Acknowledge what my experience was; it's
not yours to accept or dismiss.

It's yours to acknowledge as my experience.

This is my story. My pain. My hurt.

See me for who I am, and for what happened to me.

This is how I heal,
when others stop denying my reality and,
instead, acknowledge and respect it.

DID I JUST FEEL
SAFE IN MY BODY?

YOU WILL—FOR NO PARTICULAR REASON—NOTICE one day that you feel okay. That is the moment you start to feel safe in your body. It is a homecoming. It feels like you might want to do something! It feels like a world of possibilities. Curiosity and excitement arrive.

It feels as if being alone is okay now. It feels as if you can go to the movies, and that being by yourself is good, perhaps even better than dealing with others. It feels strong and innate inside. It is like discovering a landscape of safety inside of you. Your old thoughts can still come in, and you might—for a second—start to feel that old fear. That is okay.

Your nervous system is just pulling you back to the old state of preparation and readiness , where you have been for decades. Safety can be perceived by your survival brain as dangerous, because it is new and different. Notice and acknowledge that protection mechanism in yourself, and then come back to safety. Even if you stay there for only twenty seconds, what a delicious moment to feel again.

Welcome it. It is your victory. Celebrate it. It will not dissipate. It will be minimized, and it may be absent for a couple of days, but the moment you start to feel safe in your body, there is no going back. You will feel it more and more, and it will keep growing.

It is a precious moment in your healing journey. Notice and savor all these micro-victories. Feeling this way is monumental and a long time coming. Congratulations.

SAYING NO

THE MOMENT YOU STAND UP FOR YOURSELF WHEN someone is condescending toward you, you will feel an innate power inside. You will feel strong and proud, and even better, you will survive it.

The judgmental, timid voice inside your head will quiet for the first time. That silence means your inner child feels protected and is proud of you! Your inner self-judging voice suddenly has full respect for you. The adult you.

When you learn that you are an adult who needs to speak up in order not to be dismissed or ridiculed—even if it's uncomfortable—your strength will return, and the critical voices in your head will quiet. Your posture will change, and your dignity will be restored.

Saying "No," or "Enough," or "Hell no you won't!" can cause an internal shift on so many levels.

You will feel like an adult. The submissive, obedient part of you will feel so protected and proud, and you will learn that you have the ability to take care of yourself. You don't need to wait for a prince to protect you.

The need for a savior is the core of codependency, which manifests as powerlessness and a loss of agency. Waiting for your partner, your parent, or anyone to protect you makes you a victim. That waiting comes from the child who is frozen inside of you, waiting to be rescued by a parent who clearly never showed up and sadly, never will.

The fact is, you are now an adult who needs to come out of that childhood freeze-response and learn to say no. Saying no is never easy for anyone.

Your no doesn't have to be defensive, or justifying, or delivered with rage. It can be clear, precise, strong or soft, and simple. Just a quick, "No, you can't," and then go back to your business.

You're not left hanging, not forced to justify your no or waiting around for some douchebag to decide for you. No, that would be submission. You didn't wait; you decided, said no, and continued on with your day. It will feel awkward and scary at first, but the delicious strength you will gain will help you to come back into your adult self and finally grow up.

There is no prince or knight in shining armor who will do this work for you. Even a knight gets tired, or overworked, and needs time to rest, away from everyone. Your job is to take full responsibility and learn how to stand up for yourself, and learn that saying no to douchebags will not be your death sentence.

However, please do not do this if you are in a violent relationship. If you are in a violent relationship, please find the resources and support you need to protect yourself first.

Learning to stand up for yourself and say no—in a safe environment—will become your first pathway to independence, adulthood, and the fullness of your own being. Welcome home.

WHY DOES SHE LOOK BETTER THAN US?

AFTER YEARS OF BEING DEPRIVED, YOUR INNER CHILD feels safe and understands you are a protective adult. This will allow them to be exuberant, enthusiastic, free, and optimistic, just like before the trauma happened. That child in us goes back to their innate, vital state.

The moment you start to feel safe inside of yourself and your environment, the wonder and joy of your vital energy will rush and move through you, out and into the world. People will question why you are so vibrant, content, at peace, and energized.

They will say, "She changed," or "You look different somehow." They will wonder, *Wasn't she abused? Isn't she supposed to hide from the world and be broken?*

Well, quite the opposite is happening in your nervous system, once you come through to the other side of the veil. Post-traumatic growth is happening, and the force of your oppressed life energy finally gets to take space and flourish. Thrive! Enjoy it. Use it. This quality will never be taken from you again. May the force finally be with you!

YOUR POWER

PEOPLE OFTEN ASSOCIATE POWER WITH SOMETHING outside of them, or what is done to them. Quite often, power is coupled with harm, violence, submission, obedience.

The truth about power is that it resides in you. It has internal, witnessing eyes. That power is best described as trust. It is the quality of trusting yourself, your being, your presence, your mind, and your body. It is the vast space of knowing. It is the abundance of trust. It is soft. It is a space of boundless intelligence, presence, and monumental strength—not force—but the strength of the largest mountains.

In that space, you don't doubt yourself or your experience, nor do you question yourself. It is a place where tenderness, strength, and resiliency merge. You are clear enough to receive and read all of the cues of your proprioception, your environment, and your interoception, of how your body is responding.

Your body syncs with the space in which you rest. Your environment also becomes an extension of your inner space. That is when you notice someone entering a restaurant, or a boardroom, and seeming so comfortable, so at ease in their skin. That is innate power, that is a person's essence.

We all have it. We are born with innate power. It is passed down from our ancestors, thousands of years of power collected and stored in us. Then, at some point in our life, it was dismissed, destroyed, and distorted by the domination that we associate with power in the modern world.

You do not need to spend money, go on retreats, or do plant medicine to find it again. Simply start with one minute of meditation a day, or pray, or do any repetitive manual task such as knitting or walking, and notice that subliminal quiet power arising within you. Usually, it sits in your midline, at the back of your spine. Tap into that. It is very simple, deep, and accessible. It is in you.

HOLDING SPACE

TO HOLD SPACE FOR YOURSELF MEANS TO HAVE THE capacity to hold what arises inside of you. In that moment of witnessing and holding, you observe your emotion, your experience, and your state. In holding space, there is no judgment, blaming, or justifying; there is only pure witnessing of the self.

This space is a place where your innate intelligence, ancestral wisdom, and grace meet. It is a vast space in which healing starts. It resides in you, and in those who know how to witness your experience, your truth. They are good listeners. They are holders of space. You might hold space for others, but you haven't yet developed the ability to hold space for yourself.

Surround yourself with people who can hold space for you, and you will start to mirror that back. Listen to yourself as if someone was listening to you. This is what your therapist is doing for you. Any skilled therapist will develop those capabilities inside of you.

When you learn to hold your own space, you can finally notice and name what you feel and what you need. You will take enough time and space to process, and to decide what is and is not okay for you.

SELF-VALIDATION

THE TRAUMA MIND SEEKS VALIDATION FROM THE person who hurt us. That validation will never come. It is a fantasy that you need to awaken from. Prince Charming is not coming, and neither is a mature parent capable of self-reflection. If you need to seek validation from the outside, find someone who was in your shoes, someone who has the capacity and intelligence to see you.

True healing and coming to yourself is the result of self-validation. It needs to come from within you. Self-validation is a delicate process in healing, but it is accessible. It waits only for you to start. You do not need to wait for anyone else.

When you validate your integrity, your experiences, your feelings, your senses, your wants, and your needs, then your self-esteem and the trust you have in yourself will expand and blossom. Drop by drop, this is golden nourishment and care for your soul—something you never got from your parents or your partner.

In neglectful or abusive relationships, you don't receive any validation of your feelings, reality, accomplishments, experiences, or needs. It is the opposite. Neglect and abuse distort your reality and invalidate anything that comes from inside of you.

"No, you are not sick."

"No, it wasn't like that."

"No, you didn't say that."

"No, that wasn't what happened."

"No, she is not a good person."

"No, you are wrong."

"That idea is ridiculous."

Do these sound familiar? It is all about dismissing, minimizing, gaslighting, and invalidating what is inside of you.

That causes you to start doubting yourself and lose trust in what is happening to you. It is insidious and crazy-making. So, start today, every hour, with validating your experiences and feelings. It sounds so trivial from the outside, yet it is the essence of bringing you back to your own reality after abuse.

You start by naming how you feel. I feel anxious. I feel hungry. I feel cold. I made this well. I love this song. I feel strong. I feel weak. I experienced anger. I was restless. I need a rest. I prefer tea. I, I, I, I.... Notice and name what you feel in the first person. Trust and value it. It is yours.

Then, you learn to communicate it to others, and if they want to distort what you're saying, who cares? You trust your experience, you validate it, and you value it. No one gets to distort your reality!

SIGNS OF HEALING

WHEN YOU REFLECT BACK ON YOUR TRAUMA AND find humor in it, it is a sign of healing. For me as a therapist, it is a profound experience to witness a person who went through the unspeakable, and who still has the ability to find a thread of humor in it.

It is like the heaviness of doom lifts and the burden of that trauma becomes lighter. Humor is cathartic in the healing process. It brings a sense of greater ease. The birthplace of the most brilliant humor is in trauma survivors. If you want someone to write excellent comedies and stand-ups, hire a trauma survivor.

Nothing births humor in people like the pain of trauma and PTSD.

VICTIM LABELS

DID YOUR ABUSER AND THE PATRIARCHAL SYSTEM IN which you lived label victimhood as shameful, all so they could excuse their bad behavior? It's almost humiliating to acknowledge you're a victim, and to truly know you have been wronged. Look at Hollywood. Victims are endemic in Tinsel Town, and no one is saying anything but, "I am not a victim!" or "I don't want to be called a victim."

Perhaps the producers and moguls who were assaulting young children and sexually exploiting the entire industry said, "Don't play the victim," so they could get away with it. They turned saying, "I am a victim," into a badge of shame.

It's a belief imposed by the perpetrators for their benefit.

"Oh, she's playing the victim." Yes, some people pretend to be victims, but that isn't common. The cultural shaming and silencing of victims makes them stay quiet. Isn't that exactly what the assailants want?

When I hear clients say, "I am not a victim," I say to them, "So, you just gave a free pass and zero accountability to someone who assaulted you; is this justice for you? This is advocating for the abuser, not yourself. You are advocating for everyone who shames victims."

"You are playing the victim," is what every predator who wants a free pass with his prey says.

Victims need to respond to these predators. "You can trivialize what you did by saying I am playing the victim," they might say, "but being dehumanized is not a play or a line from a script. I have been victimized by your behavior. I *am* a victim. You will be accountable for it and you will face justice. Society will also cast judgment, and I am not giving you a free pass."

Feel those words. There is no playing the victim here. Here is a human standing up for what has been done to them, standing up for the victim they have been in that perpetrator's hands. If that is not agency and bravery, what is?

Own it. Stand up and say you are a victim. And never give a free pass to someone who slaps the "playing the victim" label onto others, allowing them to remain free while continuing their abuse.

FROM SADNESS TO SORROW TO NEW POWER

WHEN YOU FACE ALL THAT HAPPENED AND ALL THE losses you encountered, acceptance will settle in your body and sadness will show up. Welcome your sadness. You can finally begin your healing process. A mourning dance will move you forward to more peaceful days.

I danced with my sorrow for a very long t me, for as long as I needed. Sorrow is prolonged sadness. It is a vulnerable, graceful, soft, fragile, and sacred place to be in your trauma recovery. It is a place where emptiness shows up and resets your mind, soul, and body.

The body craves sadness. It wants to fina ly sit down and rest and mourn with the heart. The mind never allows it. The mind wants to pull you out of sorrow and keep fighting. It doesn't want to acknowledge the losses, to break family loyalty, to say the necessary goodbyes to the people who hurt you. The mind wants pretense. The body wants authenticity.

When you allow it, sadness will come into your body as a fresh breeze after the turmoil of your exper ences. Sadness will let you finally take a peaceful breath, expand, and show up wise and full of strength. It will feel like you are becoming a new person. Soft power will rise from you, but do not confuse the word soft with being incapable or less than.

The soft power that emerges has a depth of resiliency, the innate awareness of your story, and what you have been through. You will stand in your power once you welcome sadness.

WITH A THERAPIST

In a graceful holding, I witnessed all my grief.

In tender inquiry, my tears found release.

In a pregnant pause, I started to feel.

In a relational space, relief showed on my face.

In that supportive field, I leaned back and took a breath.

In witnessing the kindness of your
eyes, trust finally arrived.

In your accepting arms, I saw the
rebirth of a beautiful smile.

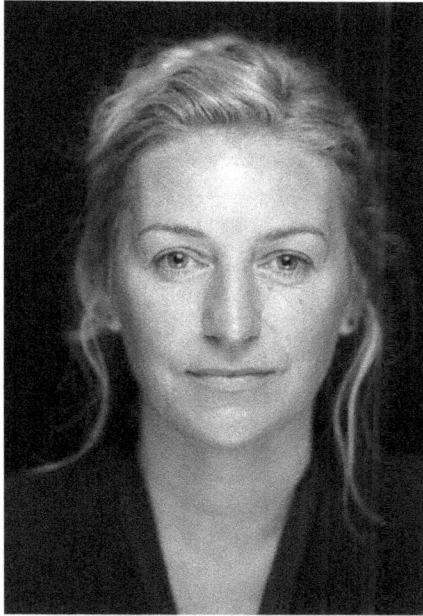

NEXT STEPS

Sign up for my newsletter to gain an early preview to Trauma We Don't Talk About series and be the first to discover my upcoming projects, events, and other news. Let's stay connected and continue to talk.

anamael.com/news

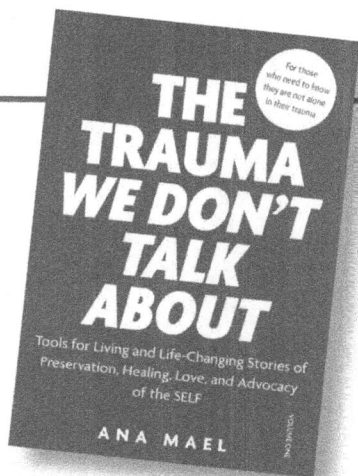

Thank you for reading
The Trauma We Don't Talk About

Would you be willing to help spread the word?

If you recognize yourself or someone you care about in even one of the essays in this book, please share it with others and leave a review anywhere you go to find and discuss good books. Sharing and reviewing The Trauma We Don't Talk About increases the number of people who find it on platforms. The more positive feedback the book receives, the more people will talk about what trauma is and how we can help each other heal. It is worth reviewing and sharing with those who believe they are alone in their trauma.

To write your review, please go to:

anamael.com/review

NOTES FOR
SELF

_____

_____

_____

_____

_____

_____

_____

_____

_____

_____

_____

_____

_____

_____

_____

www.ingramcontent.com/pod-product-compliance
Lightning Source LLC
Chambersburg PA
CBHW070615030426
42337CB00020B/3811